Gut Wisdom

The Essential Guide to a Balanced Digestive System

by

Carlos P. Branch

Disclaimer

The content provided in "Gut Wisdom: The Essential Guide to a Balanced Digestive System" is for informational purposes only and is not intended as medical advice, diagnosis, or treatment. The information contained in this book is based on research, personal experiences, and the knowledge of the authors. However, it is not a substitute for professional medical advice, diagnosis, or treatment.

Always seek the advice of your physician or other qualified health providers with any questions you may have regarding a medical condition or the use of dietary supplements, dietary changes, or lifestyle modifications. Never disregard professional medical advice or delay in seeking it because of something you have read in this book.

The authors and publishers of "Gut Wisdom: The Essential Guide to a Balanced Digestive System" are not responsible for any adverse effects or consequences resulting from the use of any suggestions, preparations, or procedures discussed in this book. The reader assumes full responsibility for any actions taken based on the information provided herein.

Individual results may vary, and the effectiveness of any recommendations, including dietary and lifestyle changes, will depend on various factors, including but not limited to individual health conditions, genetics, and adherence to the suggested guidelines.

By reading this book, you acknowledge that you understand and agree to this disclaimer. If you have any health concerns or conditions, it is always best to consult with a healthcare professional before making any significant changes to your diet, exercise routine, or health practices.

Table of contents

Introduction..7
   Welcome to Gut Wisdom..................................... 7
   The significance of gut health........................... 8
   How to Use This Book:...................................... 11

Chapter 1..15
Understanding the Gut..15
   Anatomy of the Digestive System...................... 15
   The microbiome is your inner ecosystem............. 19
   The Gut-Brain Connection: How Your Gut Influences Your Mind..22

Chapter 2..26
Common Gut Issues and Symptoms.......................26
   Digestive Disorders: Causes and Symptoms......... 26
   Recognize the signs of an unhealthy gut...............30
   The Effects of Stress on Digestion....................... 34

Chapter 3..38
Nutrition for a Healthy Gut......................................38
   The Importance of Diet in Gut Health................... 38
   Gut-Friendly Foods: What to Eat......................... 41
   Food to Avoid: What to Cut Back On....................44

Chapter 4..48
Probiotics and Prebiotics... 48
   Understanding Probiotics: Healthy Bacteria for Your Gut..48
   The benefits of prebiotics: feeding your gut bacteria..

51

Incorporating probiotics and prebiotics in your diet 54

Chapter 5 58

Lifestyle Changes to Improve Digestion 58

The importance of hydration 58

Exercise and gut health 61

Sleep and its impact on digestion 64

Chapter 6 68

Heal and Restore Your Gut 68

Identifying Food Sensitivity and Allergies 68

Detoxify your gut 70

Natural remedies and supplements 73

Chapter 7 77

The Mind-Gut Connection 77

How Stress Impacts Your Gut 77

Mindfulness and meditation for gut health 80

Strategies for managing stress 82

Chapter 8 86

Personalized Gut Health Plans 87

Creating a Gut Health Journal 87

Tailoring your diet and lifestyle 91

Chapter 9 97

Recipes for Gut Health 98

Breakfasts: Starting Your Day Right 98

Lunches: Midday Gut Boosters 104

Dinners: Evening Digestive Support 109

Snacks and Smoothies: Quick and Healthy Options.. 115

Chapter 10 119

Case Studies and Success Stories......................... 119
    Real-Life Transformations....................... 119
    Expert insights and advice..................... 123
    Lessons Learned and Key Takeaways................ 125

Conclusion... 129
    Recap of Key Points............................. 130
    Encouragement and Motivation for Your Gut Health Journey... 136
    Additional resources and references.................... 139

Appendices.. 143

Introduction

Welcome to Gut Wisdom.

Welcome to "Gut Wisdom: The Essential Guide to a Balanced Digestive System." Whether you're just starting to investigate the complexity of gut health or looking to expand your knowledge, this book is intended to be your thorough guide on the path to optimal digestive health.

In recent years, gut health has emerged as an important area of concern for both medical experts and individuals looking to enhance their overall health. The digestive system, also known as the "second brain," is crucial to our physical and mental health. However, for many, the complexities of gut health remain a mystery. This book seeks to demystify the subject, giving you practical information and real ways to improve your gut health.

You may ask why gut health has received so much attention. The explanation is simple: a healthy gut is essential for a healthy body and mind. From nutrition absorption and immunological function to mental clarity and emotional balance, your gut health has an impact on almost every area of your well-being. This book will walk you through understanding your gut, identifying indicators of imbalance, and adopting measures to build a strong digestive system.

As you embark on this adventure, remember to approach it with curiosity and openness. Gut health is more than just avoiding discomfort; it's about caring for a fundamental part of yourself that has a substantial impact on your quality of life. The chapters that follow contain a wealth of information designed to help you attain a healthy and thriving gut.

The significance of gut health

Gut health is an extremely important topic that goes far beyond the occasional stomach upset or digestive discomfort. The gut, often known as the gastrointestinal tract (GI), is a complex system that is essential for overall health. To completely understand its value, let's look at some crucial aspects:

1. Nutrient Absorption:
The gut's principal role is to digest and absorb nutrients. Every cell in your body depends on nutrients from your

diet to function properly. When your gut is healthy, it effectively digests food and absorbs necessary vitamins, minerals, and other nutrients, nourishing your body and supporting all of its activities. A damaged stomach, on the other hand, can cause malabsorption, which can lead to deficiencies that influence many aspects of health, including energy levels and immunological function.

2. Immunosystem Support:
The gut contains a large amount of your immune system. The gut-associated lymphoid tissue (GALT) includes a huge number of immune cells that fight infections. A healthy gut microbiome—the community of bacteria that live in your intestines—plays an important role in controlling immune responses. An imbalance in gut bacteria can cause immunological dysregulation, increasing vulnerability to infections and autoimmune diseases.

3. Mental Health:
The gut-brain axis is a bidirectional communication network that connects the gut to the brain. The neurological system, immunological system, and gut bacteria all play roles in facilitating this relationship. New research reveals that gut health has a substantial impact on mental health issues like anxiety, sadness, and stress. For example, gut bacteria strongly impact the creation of neurotransmitters such as serotonin, also known as the "happy hormone."

4. Inflammation and Chronic Disease:
Chronic inflammation is the underlying cause of many modern diseases, including heart disease, diabetes, and some malignancies. The gut microbiota helps to modulate inflammatory reactions. Dysbiosis, or an imbalance in the gut microbiota, can result in increased intestinal permeability (also known as "leaky gut"), allowing toxins and pathogens to enter the circulation and cause systemic inflammation.

5. Weight Management:
Gut health is closely related to metabolism and weight management. Certain gut bacteria influence how we store fat, control blood sugar, and react to hunger hormones. An imbalance in gut bacteria can lead to weight gain and metabolic problems like obesity and type 2 diabetes.

6. Detoxification:
The gut plays an important function in detoxifying the body. Regular bowel movements help to eliminate waste products and poisons. A healthy stomach promotes efficient detoxification processes, whereas an unhealthy gut can lead to toxin buildup, negatively impacting health.

Given these vital responsibilities, it is evident that preserving gut health is essential not only for preventing digestive disorders but also for general health. Investing in your gut health can significantly increase your quality of life, energy, mental clarity, and lifespan.

How to Use This Book:

"Gut Wisdom: The Essential Guide to a Balanced Digestive System" is designed to give you a complete understanding of gut health, practical guidance, and specific methods for achieving and maintaining a balanced digestive system. Here's how to get the most out of this book:

1. Start with the basics:
If you're new to the concept of gut health, start with the fundamental chapters. These sections cover the anatomy of the digestive system, the gut microbiota, and the gut-brain relationship. Understanding the fundamentals will provide you with a firm platform to build on as you go deeper into the subject.

2. Identify and address gut issues.
The chapters on common gut disorders and symptoms will assist you in recognizing the signs of an unhealthy gut. These sections cover a variety of digestive problems, their causes, and symptoms. By recognizing particular difficulties, you can personalize your approach to meet your own gut health requirements.

3. Implement nutritional strategies.
Nutrition is a critical component of intestinal health. Dietary chapters contain thorough information on gut-friendly and avoidable foods. You'll learn the benefits of probiotics and prebiotics, as well as how to incorporate them into your diet. Use the meal plans and recipes supplied to start nourishing your gut right away.

4. Adopt lifestyle changes.
Beyond diet, lifestyle factors like hydration, exercise, and sleep are important for gut health. The chapters on lifestyle modifications provide practical advice for implementing healthy behaviors into your daily life. These sections underline the need to take a comprehensive approach to gut health, taking into account all aspects of your lifestyle.

5. Explore Healing and Restorative Practices:
For people suffering from serious gut health difficulties, the healing and restoration chapters offer ways for cleaning the gut, recognizing dietary sensitivities, and employing natural therapies and supplements. These portions are especially helpful for treating chronic gastrointestinal issues and restoring equilibrium.

6. Understand the mind-gut connection.
Stress and mental wellness are closely related to gut health. The chapters on the mind-gut link look at how stress affects digestion and propose stress-management

approaches like mindfulness, meditation, and other practices. By addressing both the mind and the gut, you may take a more holistic approach to wellness.

7. Personalize your gut health plan.
Everyone's intuition is unique, so what works for one person may not work for another. The chapters on tailored gut health plans will show you how to start a gut health journal, tailor your food and lifestyle, and establish long-term strategies for gut health. This tailored approach means that you can tailor the advice to your specific needs.

8. Learn from real-life examples.
The case studies and success stories offer inspiration and practical advice from people who have successfully improved their gut health. These real-life examples demonstrate the transformative power of the tactics presented in the book and provide inspiration for your path.

9. Utilize Additional Resources:
The appendices contain a glossary of words, suggested reading, and helpful websites and support groups. These resources are intended to provide you with further knowledge and assistance as you research and improve your gut health.

10. Stay engaged and motivated.

Gut health is an ongoing process, not a one-time treatment. Revisit the chapters on a regular basis, update your gut health notebook, and remain up-to-date on new research and advancements in the field. The more you study and apply, the more advantages you will gain.

By following these suggestions, you can maximize the benefits of "gut wisdom" and embark on a revolutionary path to a healthier, more balanced digestive system. Remember that enhancing your gut health is an investment in your overall well-being, which will lead to a happier, healthier lifestyle.

This book is more than just a collection of facts; it's a road map for greater health. Approach it with an open mind, a willingness to learn, and a determination to effect positive change. Your gut—and your entire body—will appreciate you for it.

Chapter 1

Understanding the Gut.

Anatomy of the Digestive System

To truly appreciate the complexity of gut health, one must first understand the structure and function of the digestive system. This system, which breaks down food, absorbs nutrients, and excretes waste, is made up of multiple interrelated organs, each of which plays an important part in overall health.

1. Mouth:
Digestion occurs in the mouth, where mechanical and chemical processes start the breakdown of food. Chewing physically breaks down food into tiny pieces, increasing the surface area for enzymes to work on. The salivary glands create saliva, which contains amylase, an enzyme that begins the digestion of carbohydrates.

2. Esophagus:
When food is chewed and combined with saliva, it forms a bolus that is swallowed and passed down the esophagus. The esophagus is a muscular tube that links the neck and stomach. Peristaltic motions are wave-like muscular contractions that drive the bolus towards the stomach.

3. Stomach:
The stomach is a muscular, J-shaped organ that functions as a temporary storage and mixing chamber for meals. Gastric fluids, which contain hydrochloric acid and digestive enzymes such as pepsin, continue to break down proteins. The stomach's acidic environment also aids in the elimination of dangerous microorganisms and the activation of specific enzymes. The food is converted into a semi-liquid substance known as chyme.

4. Small intestine:
The small intestine is a lengthy, coiled tube where the majority of digestion and nutrient absorption take place. It is made up of three sections: the duodenum, jejunum, and ileum. The pancreas releases digestive enzymes, and the liver releases bile into the duodenum, which aids in the digestion of fats, proteins, and carbohydrates. The small intestine walls are lined with villi and microvilli, which are tiny finger-like projections that increase the surface area available for absorption. Nutrients move through these structures and into the bloodstream.

5. Pancreas, liver, and gallbladder:
These additional organs perform critical roles in digestion. The pancreas secretes digesting enzymes and bicarbonate, which neutralize stomach acid in the small intestine. The liver produces bile, which is necessary for fat digestion and is stored in the gallbladder before being released into the small intestine as needed. The liver also

digests foods absorbed through the small intestine, detoxifies toxic compounds, and stores vitamins and minerals.

6. Large intestine:
The large intestine, often known as the colon, absorbs water and electrolytes from indigestible food and produces solid waste. It is made up of the cecum, colon, rectum, and anal canal. The large intestine is home to a wide colony of bacteria that further digest specific fibers, resulting in beneficial short-chain fatty acids and vitamins.

7. Rectus and Anus:
The rectum retains feces until they are released from the body via the anus during defecation. Muscles are contracted in a coordinated manner, and sphincters are relaxed.

Each component of the digestive system works together to guarantee proper digestion and nutrition absorption while also protecting the body from dangerous bacteria and toxins.

The microbiome is your inner ecosystem.

The gut microbiome, or "inner ecosystem," is a complex and dynamic population of billions of microorganisms that live mostly in the large intestine. This community contains bacteria, viruses, fungi, and other microorganisms that are essential for maintaining health and equilibrium. Diet, environment, genetics, and lifestyle all have an impact on the human microbiome, which is distinct for each individual.

1. Composition of the gut microbiome:
The gut microbiome is extremely varied, including thousands of distinct microbial species. The microbiome composition varies throughout the gastrointestinal system. The stomach, due to its acidic environment, has fewer bacteria than the intestines. The small intestine has a moderate amount of bacteria, whereas the big intestine is highly populated with germs.

2. Functions of the Gut Microbiome:
Digestion and Nutrient Absorption: The gut microbiota helps break down complex carbohydrates, fibers, and other indigestible components. It creates enzymes that human cells do not have, which aid in the digestion of these substances and improve nutritional absorption.
Vitamin Production: Certain gut bacteria produce vital vitamins, including vitamin K and various B vitamins, which are absorbed by the host.
Immune System Regulation: The gut microbiota stimulates immune cell growth and function. It helps the body distinguish between harmful pathogens and good bacteria, thereby preventing infections and autoimmune

illnesses.

Metabolism and Energy Production: Gut bacteria convert undigested fibers into short-chain fatty acids (SCFAs) such as acetate, propionate, and butyrate. SCFAs provide energy to colon cells while also influencing metabolism and inflammation throughout the body.

Pathogen Protection: The microbiome protects the gut lining from pathogenic microorganisms by competing for nutrition and attachment sites, creating antimicrobial chemicals, and boosting the immune response.

3. Factors influencing the gut microbiome:

Diet: The sort of diet you consume has a substantial impact on the gut microbiome's composition and diversity. Diets heavy in fiber, fruits, vegetables, and fermented foods support a healthy microbiome, whereas diets high in processed foods, sugar, and fat can cause dysbiosis (microbial imbalance).

Antibiotics and medications: Antibiotics can disturb the gut microbiome's equilibrium by killing beneficial bacteria, perhaps leading to an overgrowth of dangerous germs. Other medications that can impact the microbiome include proton pump inhibitors and nonsteroidal anti-inflammatory drugs.

Lifestyle Factors: Stress, sleep, exercise, and exposure to toxins all have an impact on the gut flora. Chronic stress, for example, can influence gut bacterial makeup and function.

Age and Genetics: The gut microbiome evolves over time, from infancy to old age. Genetic factors influence the microbiome's makeup and function.

4. Gut microbiome and health:

Digestive Health: Maintaining digestive health requires a balanced gut flora, which helps to prevent illnesses like irritable bowel syndrome (IBS), inflammatory bowel disease (IBD), and celiac.

Metabolic Health: The microbiome has an impact on metabolism and energy balance, potentially increasing the risk of obesity, type 2 diabetes, and metabolic syndrome.

Mental Health: New research reveals a substantial link between the gut microbiome and mental health, which influences mood, behavior, and cognitive performance.

Immunological Health: The microbiota regulates immunological responses, thereby reducing infections, allergies, and autoimmune illnesses.

Maintaining a healthy gut flora is critical for overall health and wellness. This can be accomplished by eating a well-balanced diet, exercising regularly, managing stress, and using antibiotics and drugs responsibly.

The Gut-Brain Connection: How Your Gut Influences Your Mind.

The gut-brain connection is a bidirectional communication network that connects the gastrointestinal tract and the brain. This complex link is mediated by neurological, hormonal, and immunological processes known together as the gut-brain axis. Understanding this relationship exposes how gut health affects mental health and vice versa.

1. Neural Pathways:
The vagus nerve is the principal neurological channel that connects the gut to the brain. It sends information from the gut to the brain and vice versa, affecting motility, secretion, and inflammation. Vagal tone, or the activity of the vagus nerve, is linked to the body's ability to regulate stress and maintain homeostasis.
Enteric Nervous System (ENS): Known as the "second brain," the ENS is a network of neurons buried in the intestinal wall. It functions autonomously but communicates with the CNS to regulate digestion processes and respond to gut inputs.

2. Hormonal Pathways:
Gut Hormones: The gut generates a variety of hormones that control hunger, digestion, and fullness, including ghrelin, cholecystokinin (CCK), and peptide

YY (PYY). These hormones affect mood and behavior by acting on the brain.

Neurotransmitters: The gut microbiome synthesizes and regulates neurotransmitters such as serotonin, dopamine, and gamma-aminobutyric acid. Serotonin, also known as the "happy hormone," is produced predominantly in the gut and plays an important role in mood control.

3. Immune pathways:

Immune Modulation: The gut microbiota communicates with the immune system, affecting the production of cytokines and other immune mediators. These chemicals can influence brain function and behavior, connecting gut health to immune responses and neuroinflammation.

4. Psychological and behavioral effects:

Mood Disorders: Dysbiosis in the gut microbiome has been linked to mood problems like despair and anxiety. Gut bacteria can change the production of neurotransmitters and inflammatory indicators, affecting brain function and mood.

Stress Response: Chronic stress can alter the gut flora, causing increased intestinal permeability (leaky gut) and systemic inflammation. This, in turn, influences brain function and stress resilience.

Cognitive Function: A new study indicates that the gut microbiome affects cognitive processes like memory, learning, and decision-making. Alterations in gut microbes have been linked to cognitive decline and neurodegenerative disorders.

5. Therapeutic implications:
Probiotics and Prebiotics: Adding probiotics (beneficial microorganisms) and prebiotics (fiber that

Feeding beneficial microorganisms can enhance gut health and potentially reduce symptoms of mood disorders and cognitive problems.

Dietary Interventions: Consuming fiber, polyphenols, and omega-3 fatty acids promotes a healthy gut flora and may improve mental health. Fermented foods such as yogurt, kefir, and sauerkraut are natural sources of probiotics.

Mindfulness and Stress Management: Meditation, yoga, and deep breathing can all improve vagal tone and support a healthy gut-brain connection. Reducing stress can improve gut health and general well-being.

The gut-brain connection emphasizes the necessity of taking a holistic approach to health, acknowledging that mental and physical health are inextricably linked. Individuals can improve their overall health and resilience by nurturing both their gut and mind.

Chapter 2

Common Gut Issues and Symptoms.

Digestive Disorders: Causes and Symptoms

Digestive disorders are a group of illnesses that affect the gastrointestinal (GI) tract, resulting in discomfort, abnormal bowel habits, and other systemic symptoms. Understanding the origins and symptoms of these illnesses is critical for successful gut health management. Here, we look at several common digestive diseases, their causes, and symptoms.

1. Gastroesophageal reflux disorder (GERD):
Causes: GERD develops when stomach acid repeatedly rushes back into the esophagus, irritating its lining. A weak lower esophageal sphincter (LES), obesity, pregnancy, smoking, and certain meals and beverages can all play a role.
Common symptoms include heartburn, regurgitation of

food or sour fluids, chest pain, difficulty swallowing, chronic cough, laryngitis, and sleep disturbances.

2. Irritable Bowel Syndrome:
Causes: Although the specific etiology of IBS is unknown, it is believed to be a mix of aberrant gut motility, visceral hypersensitivity, and psychosocial factors. Stress, hormonal fluctuations, specific diets, and gastrointestinal diseases are all potential triggers.
Symptoms: Symptoms may include abdominal pain or cramping, bloating, gas, diarrhea, constipation, or an alternating combination of the two. Symptoms may be chronic and fluctuate in severity.

3. Inflammatory Bowel Disorder (IBD):
Causes: IBD refers to chronic inflammatory disorders of the gastrointestinal system, most notably Crohn's disease and ulcerative colitis. The specific etiology is unknown, although it is associated with an aberrant immune response to gut bacteria that is controlled by genetic and environmental factors.
Symptoms: Crohn's disease can affect any section of the gastrointestinal tract, causing abdominal pain, diarrhea (sometimes bloody), weight loss, exhaustion, and malnutrition. Ulcerative colitis affects the colon and rectum, creating chronic inflammation and ulceration, resulting in stomach pain, bloody diarrhea, and the need to defecate.

4. Celiac Disease:
Causes: Celiac disease is an autoimmune illness caused by gluten (a protein present in wheat, barley, and rye). Gluten ingestion in celiac disease patients causes immune-mediated damage to the small intestine.
Symptoms: Symptoms might range from diarrhea, bloating, gas, lethargy, weight loss, anemia, and nutrient malabsorption. Some people may develop non-gastrointestinal symptoms such as dermatitis herpetiformis (a skin rash), joint pain, and neurological problems.

5. Diverticular Diseases:
Causes: Diverticular disease results in the creation of tiny bulging pouches (diverticula) in the colon wall. It is assumed to be the result of increased intestinal pressure, which could be caused by a low-fiber diet, constipation, or age.
Symptoms: Many patients with diverticula have no symptoms (diverticulosis). When the diverticula become inflamed or infected (diverticulitis), symptoms may include stomach pain (usually on the lower left side), fever, nausea, vomiting, and changes in bowel patterns.

6. Small intestinal bacterial overgrowth (SIBO):
Causes: SIBO develops when too many bacteria inhabit the small intestine, which generally has fewer bacteria than the large intestine. Impairment of intestinal motility, anatomical abnormalities, and illnesses such as diabetes,

scleroderma, and prior abdominal surgery are all potential causes.

Symptoms may include bloating, stomach pain, diarrhea, constipation, malabsorption, and vitamin deficiencies. SIBO can mirror the symptoms of other intestinal illnesses, making diagnosis difficult.

7. Gallstones:

Causes: Gallstones are solid particles formed in the gallbladder from cholesterol, bilirubin, and bile salts. Obesity, quick weight reduction, particular diets, and genetic susceptibility all pose risks.

Symptoms: Many people who have gallstones show no symptoms. However, when a gallstone plugs a bile duct, it can cause severe discomfort in the upper right abdomen, nausea, vomiting, and perhaps jaundice (yellowing of the skin and eyes).

Understanding these digestive problems aids in diagnosing and treating symptoms early on, allowing for proper medical intervention and management.

Recognize the signs of an unhealthy gut.

An unhealthy gut can show a range of signs and symptoms, many of which point to underlying digestive issues. Recognizing these symptoms is the first step in treating gut health issues and obtaining appropriate treatment. Here are some frequent symptoms of an unhealthy gut:

1. Digestive discomfort:
Bloating: Persistent bloating may indicate an imbalance in gut bacteria, poor digestion, or dietary intolerances.
Gas: Excess gas can be caused by the bacterial fermentation of undigested food in the intestines.
Abdominal discomfort: Recurrent or chronic abdominal discomfort could suggest IBS, IBD, or SIBO.

2. Changed Bowel Habits:
Diarrhea: Frequent loose or watery stools may indicate an illness, dietary intolerance, or chronic condition such as IBS or IBD.
Constipation: Infrequent or difficult bowel movements can be caused by a low-fiber diet, dehydration, or underlying conditions like IBS.
Irregular Bowel Movements: Alternating diarrhea and constipation may suggest IBS or other digestive disorders.

3. Food intolerances and sensitivities:
Food Reactions: Symptoms such as bloating, gas, diarrhea, or stomach cramps after eating particular foods may indicate a food intolerance or sensitivity.
Common Triggers: Dairy, gluten, and certain carbohydrates (FODMAPs) are common causes.

4. Skin Issues:
Acne, Eczema, and Psoriasis: Skin problems can be connected to gut health via the gut-skin axis. Dysbiosis or leaky gut can cause systemic inflammation, which affects the skin.
Rashes and hives: Sudden skin reactions may suggest dietary allergies or intolerances.

5. Fatigue and poor sleep:
Chronic weariness: An unhealthy gut can reduce nutritional absorption, resulting in inadequacies that contribute to weariness.
Sleep disturbances: The gut creates and regulates neurotransmitters such as serotonin, which influence sleep. Gut problems might interfere with sleep habits.

6. Mood Disorders:
Anxiety and Depression: The gut-brain axis connects gut health with mental wellness. Dysbiosis and inflammation can impair neurotransmitter synthesis, leading to mood problems.
Brain Fog: Systemic inflammation and inadequate nutrient absorption can cause concentration difficulties and cognitive impairment.

7. Unexpected Weight Changes:
Weight Gain: An imbalance in gut flora can disrupt metabolism, causing weight gain or difficulties reducing weight.

Weight Loss: Chronic diarrhea, malabsorption, or illnesses such as celiac disease can cause unintentional weight loss.

8. Autoimmune Conditions:
Immune Dysregulation: A weakened gut barrier (leaky gut) can cause immune system activation and inflammation, contributing to autoimmune diseases such as rheumatoid arthritis, lupus, and multiple sclerosis.

9. Frequent infections:
Weakened Immune System: The gut houses a significant element of the immune system. Dysbiosis can impair immune systems, resulting in recurrent infections like colds, flu, and urinary tract infections.

10. Nutrient deficiencies:
Iron, Vitamin D, and B Vitamins: Poor gut health can hinder nutritional absorption, resulting in deficiencies such as weariness, muscle weakness, and anemia.

Recognizing these symptoms enables early intervention, which can prevent subsequent issues and enhance overall health.

The Effects of Stress on Digestion

Stress is a normal and often unavoidable part of modern life, yet its effects on digestion and gut health are significant. The gut-brain axis, a bidirectional communication network that connects the gut and the brain, is critical to understanding how stress affects digestion. Here, we look at how stress affects digestion and gut health:

1. Physiological Responses to Stress:
Fight-or-flight reaction: Stress triggers the body's fight-or-flight reaction, which produces stress chemicals such as adrenaline and cortisol. These hormones help the body respond to threats by shifting energy away from non-essential tasks like digesting.
Reduced Blood Flow to the Gut: Stress causes blood flow to be redirected away from the digestive organs and toward muscles and the brain, affecting digestion.
Changed Gut Motility: Stress can either accelerate or impede gut motility, resulting in symptoms such as diarrhea or constipation.

2. Impact on gut microbiota:
Dysbiosis: Chronic stress can disrupt the makeup and diversity of the gut microbiota, resulting in dysbiosis. This imbalance can worsen digestive problems and contribute to illnesses such as IBS and IBD.

Increased Pathogenic Bacteria: Stress can stimulate the growth of pathogenic bacteria, further disturbing gut balance and jeopardizing gut health.

3. Intestinal permeability:
Leaky Gut Syndrome: Stress increases intestinal permeability, allowing undigested food particles, poisons, and infections to enter the bloodstream. This causes an immunological response and systemic inflammation, which contribute to a variety of health problems, including autoimmune disorders and allergies.

4. Inflammatory response:
Chronic inflammation: Stress-induced dysbiosis and leaky gut can cause chronic inflammation.

This affects not only the gut but also other organs and systems in the body. Chronic inflammation has been related to a variety of health concerns, including metabolic abnormalities, cardiovascular diseases, and mental health issues.

5. Symptoms of Stress-Related Digestive Problems:
Heartburn and Acid Reflux: Stress can increase stomach acid production and loosen the LES, causing GERD symptoms.
Abdominal Pain and Cramping: Stress can increase pain sensitivity in the stomach, exacerbating symptoms of IBS and other functional GI diseases.

Bloating and Gas: Impaired gut motility and dysbiosis can result in increased gas production and bloating.

Diarrhea and constipation: Stress impairs gut motility, resulting in either rapid (diarrhea) or slower food transit.

6. Mental and gut health:

Anxiety and Depression: The gut-brain axis connects stress to mental health problems such as anxiety and depression. Dysbiosis and inflammation can impair the production of neurotransmitters such as serotonin and dopamine, contributing to mood disorders.

Stress and Eating Habits: Stress can influence eating habits, resulting in overeating or undereating. Emotional eating frequently includes high-calorie, low-nutrient items that exacerbate gastrointestinal health.

7. Coping Strategies and Stress Management:

Diet and Nutrition: A well-balanced diet high in fiber, fermented foods, and healthy fats promotes gut health and resilience to stress. Avoiding processed meals, sweets, and excess coffee and alcohol can help minimize intestinal inflammation.

Mindfulness and Relaxation Techniques: Meditation, yoga, deep breathing techniques, and progressive muscle relaxation can all help reduce stress and improve gut-brain communication.

Regular Physical Activity: Exercise improves gastrointestinal motility, increases blood flow to the digestive organs, and lowers stress. Choose moderate-intensity activities such as walking, cycling, or swimming.

Adequate sleep: Proper sleep is critical for general health and stress management. Poor sleep can increase stress and digestive troubles, whereas good sleep promotes the body's repair and healing mechanisms.

Social Support: Creating a strong network of friends, family, or support groups can help you manage stress and enhance your mental health.

Understanding how stress affects digestion stresses the significance of taking a comprehensive approach to gut health management. Individuals who handle stress through lifestyle modifications and mindfulness techniques can enhance their mental and intestinal health.

Chapter 3

Nutrition for a Healthy Gut

The Importance of Diet in Gut Health

Diet plays an important role in sustaining intestinal health. What you consume has a direct effect on the makeup and function of the gut microbiome, the integrity of the gut lining, and the overall efficiency of the digestive system. A gut-healthy diet can help prevent and treat a variety of digestive problems, enhance nutrition absorption, and promote overall well-being.

1. Influence on the gut microbiome:Microbial Diversity: A diverse and balanced gut microbiome is essential for overall health. Dietary variety, particularly fiber-rich plant meals, encourages microbial diversity. Different microorganisms thrive on different substrates; therefore, a varied diet promotes a diverse assortment of beneficial bacteria.Prebiotics: These non-digestible fibers contained in certain foods promote the growth and activity of beneficial bacteria. Foods high in prebiotics include garlic, onions, leeks, asparagus, bananas, and whole grains.Probiotics: These are live, helpful bacteria found in fermented foods such as yogurt, kefir, sauerkraut, kimchi, and miso. Probiotics help replace and maintain a healthy gut microbiota, which aids digestion and immunity.

2. Gut barrier function:Intestinal Permeability: The gut lining serves as a barrier, regulating what flows from the digestive tract into the bloodstream. A balanced diet can help reinforce this barrier, lowering intestinal permeability and preventing leaky gut syndrome. Nutrients such as glutamine, zinc, and omega-3 fatty acids are very important for gut health.Anti-inflammatory foods: Chronic inflammation can harm the gut lining and lead to digestive problems. Anti-inflammatory foods include fatty fish (high in omega-3 fatty acids), leafy greens, berries, nuts, and seeds, which can help reduce inflammation and promote intestinal health.

3. Digestive efficiency:Digestive Enzymes: Some meals can stimulate the production and activity of digestive enzymes. Pineapple contains bromelain, whereas papaya includes papain, both of which help with protein digestion. Fermented foods also include natural enzymes, which aid digestion.Hydration: Adequate water intake is necessary for digestion. Water aids in nutrient dissolution, absorption, and waste transit via the digestive tract.

4. Nutrient Absorption:Balanced Macronutrients: A diet rich in balanced macronutrients (carbohydrates, proteins, and fats) guarantees that the body receives a diverse variety of nutrients required for overall health and gastrointestinal function. Prioritize whole foods such as fruits and vegetables, lean meats, and healthy fats.Micronutrients: Vitamins and minerals have distinct functions in gut health. For example, vitamin D promotes gut immunological function, whereas magnesium is required for muscle activity, including digestive tract muscles.

Gut-Friendly Foods: What to Eat

Incorporating gut-friendly foods into your diet is essential for maintaining a healthy digestive tract. These nutrients promote the growth of good bacteria, reinforce the intestinal barrier, and improve overall digestion. Here are some types of gut-friendly meals, with particular examples:

1. Fiber-rich foods: Whole Grains: Brown rice, quinoa, oats, and whole wheat products are high in nutritional fiber. Fiber encourages regular bowel movements, bulks up the stool, and feeds good gut bacteria.Fruits and vegetables: apples, berries, bananas, leafy greens, broccoli, and carrots are rich in fiber and important nutrients. These foods promote a diverse microbiota and provide antioxidants that lower inflammation.

2. Fermented foods: Yogurt: Select plain, unsweetened yogurt with live, active cultures. Yogurt contains probiotics, which help balance the gut microbiota and improve digestion.Kefir is a fermented milk beverage comparable to yogurt but with a higher probiotic content. It also comes in dairy-free varieties made with coconut or almond milk.Sauerkraut and kimchi are fermented cabbage foods high in probiotics, fiber, and nutrients. They improve intestinal health and immunological function.Miso and tempeh: fermented soybean products rich in probiotics and protein. They also contain isoflavones, which have an anti-inflammatory effect.

3. Prebiotic foods: Garlic and onions are high in inulin, a form of prebiotic fiber that supports good gut bacteria. They also have antibacterial capabilities that contribute to a healthy balance of intestinal flora.Asparagus and artichokes: These plants are high in prebiotic fiber, which promotes the growth of good bacteria and improves digestive health.Bananas: In addition to being high in prebiotics, bananas are easy to digest and can help soothe upset stomachs.

4. Omega-3 Fatty Acids:Fatty Fish: Salmon, mackerel, sardines, and trout contain omega-3 fatty acids, which have anti-inflammatory properties and promote intestinal health.Chia Seeds and Flaxseeds: These plant-based omega-3 sources also contain fiber and antioxidants.

5. Polyphenol-rich foods:Berries: Blueberries, strawberries, and raspberries have high levels of polyphenols, which have antioxidant and anti-inflammatory qualities that improve gut bacteria.Green Tea: Green tea contains polyphenols, particularly catechins, which promote gut health and have anti-inflammatory properties.Dark chocolate contains flavonoids, which can benefit the gut microbiota. Choose dark chocolate with a high cocoa content (70% or greater) and few added sugars.

6. Nuts and seeds:Almonds and walnuts: Nuts are high in fiber, healthy fats, and antioxidants, which enhance gastrointestinal health and overall well-being.Pumpkin and sunflower seeds include fiber, healthy fats, and vital minerals such as magnesium and zinc, which promote gastrointestinal function and integrity.

7. Herbs and spices:Ginger: Ginger is known for its anti-inflammatory and digestive characteristics, which can help reduce nausea, stimulate digestion, and relieve bloating.Turmeric contains curcumin, a potent anti-inflammatory ingredient that promotes gut health and decreases inflammation.

Food to Avoid: What to Cut Back On

Certain foods can harm gut health by changing the microbiome, harming the gut lining, or inducing inflammation. Reducing or removing these things from your diet can help you have a healthy gut. Here are some foods and substances that should be avoided or reduced:

1. Processed food:High in Additives: Many processed foods contain artificial additives, preservatives, and colorings, which can harm gut health. These compounds can irritate the gut lining and lead to dysbiosis.Low in Nutrients: Processed foods frequently lack key nutrients and fiber, both of which are necessary for gut health. They may also include high levels of harmful fats, sugars, and processed carbs, which can disrupt the gut microbiota.

2. Sugary foods and drinks:Added sugars: Excess sugar consumption can encourage the growth of pathogenic bacteria and yeast in the gut, resulting in dysbiosis and inflammation. Sugary drinks, candies, pastries, and processed snacks are popular sources of added sugars.Artificial Sweeteners: Certain artificial sweeteners, such as aspartame and sucralose, might harm the gut microbiota. They may diminish good microorganisms and increase glucose intolerance.

3. Refined carbs:White bread and pasta: These foods lack fiber and minerals, resulting in quick blood sugar rises. They have minimal nutritional value and can upset the equilibrium of gut microbes.Pastries and Baked Goods: Because they are often manufactured with refined flour and contain a lot of sugar, they might cause gut imbalances and inflammation.

4. Fried and Fatty Foods: Trans fats, which are found in many fried and commercially baked items, have been linked to inflammation and can impair gut health. They can change the composition of the gut microbiota, increasing the risk of chronic illnesses.Greasy Foods: High-fat foods are difficult to digest and may reduce gastrointestinal motility, resulting in symptoms such as bloating and discomfort.

5. Red and processed meats:High in Saturated Fats: Red meat, particularly fatty cuts, and processed meats such as sausages and hot dogs can cause inflammation and gastrointestinal disturbances. They are also associated with an increased risk of colorectal cancer.Nitrates and Preservatives: Processed meats frequently include nitrates and other preservatives that are detrimental to gut health.

6. Dairy Products:Lactose Intolerance: Many people have difficulty digesting lactose, a sugar found in milk, which causes symptoms such as bloating, gas, and diarrhea. Lactose intolerance is more common in adulthood and in some ethnic groups.High-Fat Dairy: Full-fat dairy products can be high in saturated fats, which may cause inflammation and digestive discomfort in some people.

7. Gluten-containing foods:Gluten Sensitivity: Some people have non-celiac gluten sensitivity or celiac disease, in which gluten causes immunological reactions or digestive problems. Gluten reduction or elimination can help these people improve their intestinal health.Refined Wheat Products: Foods prepared with refined wheat flour, such as white bread and pastries, might have a negative influence on gut health due to their low fiber content and high glycemic index.

8. Alcohol: Alcohol can cause gut irritation.

irritate the gut lining, promote intestinal permeability (leaky gut), and upset the equilibrium of gut microorganisms. Excessive alcohol intake is particularly bad for intestinal health.Nutrient Absorption: Chronic alcohol use can impede nutrient absorption, leading to deficits that influence gut function and overall health.

9. Caffeine:Increases Gut Motility: Although moderate caffeine consumption may have some health benefits, excessive consumption can overstimulate the digestive tract, resulting in symptoms such as diarrhea or acid reflux.Dehydration: Caffeine is a diuretic, which causes dehydration and impairs digestion.

10. High-sodium foods:Processed Snacks and Fast Foods: A high-salt diet can disturb fluid balance in the body and harm intestinal health. It can cause bloating, hypertension, and an elevated risk of stomach cancer.

Chapter 4

Probiotics and Prebiotics.

Understanding Probiotics: Healthy Bacteria for Your Gut

Probiotics are living bacteria that offer several health benefits when ingested in sufficient quantities. They are sometimes referred to as "good" or "beneficial" bacteria because they contribute to a healthy balance in the gut microbiome, which is critical for overall health. Understanding probiotics entails studying their various kinds, mechanisms of action, and health advantages.

1. Types of probiotics: Lactobacillus: Lactobacillus is a common type of probiotic found in fermented foods and supplements. It contributes to the breakdown of lactose and the production of lactic acid, which inhibits dangerous microorganisms and improves nutritional absorption. Lactobacillus acidophilus, Lactobacillus rhamnosus, and Lactobacillus casei are three species.Bifidobacterium: These bacteria live in the intestines and are necessary for a healthy digestive tract. They aid in the digestion of dietary fiber, the production of important vitamins, and the protection against infections. Common species include Bifidobacterium bifidum, Bifidobacterium longum, and Bifidobacterium infantis.Saccharomyces boulardii: This yeast probiotic promotes gut health and has been used to treat and prevent diarrhea, particularly antibiotic-induced and traveler's diarrhea.Streptococcus thermophilus: This probiotic, which is commonly present in dairy products, aids with lactose digestion and immune system function.

2. Mechanism of Action:Colonization and Competition: Probiotics colonize the gut, competing with dangerous bacteria for nutrition and attachment sites, preventing infections from growing.Probiotics produce antimicrobial compounds such as lactic acid, hydrogen peroxide, and bacteriocins, which hinder the growth of dangerous bacteria.Gut Barrier Strengthening: Probiotics improve gut barrier function by increasing mucus and tight junction proteins, lowering intestinal permeability, and preventing leaky gut syndrome.Immune System Modulation: Probiotics interact with intestinal immune cells, increasing anti-inflammatory responses and improving the body's ability to fight infections.

3. Health Benefits of Probiotics:Digestive Health: Probiotics promote a healthy gut microbiome, which reduces symptoms of digestive illnesses like irritable bowel syndrome (IBS), inflammatory bowel disease (IBD), and diarrhea. They can also reduce constipation and bloating.Immune Function: Probiotics boost general immune function by strengthening the gut barrier and modifying immunological responses, lowering the risk of infection and autoimmune disease.Mental Health: The gut-brain axis links gut health and mental health. Probiotics can improve mood and cognitive function by lowering inflammation and regulating neurotransmitter synthesis. They have been demonstrated to reduce symptoms of anxiety, sadness, and stress.Metabolic Health: Probiotics help regulate metabolism and body weight. They can boost insulin sensitivity, lower inflammation, and aid with weight management.Skin Health: Probiotics can help with acne, eczema, and psoriasis by lowering systemic inflammation and boosting the immune system.

The benefits of prebiotics: feeding your gut bacteria

Prebiotics are nondigestible food components that stimulate the growth and activity of healthy gut bacteria. They act as food for probiotics, increasing their positive effects and promoting a healthy gut microbiota.

Understanding prebiotics entails investigating their various kinds, modes of action, and health advantages.

1. Types of Prebiotics:Fructooligosaccharides (FOS): Found in foods such as garlic, onions, bananas, and asparagus, FOS are short chains of fructose molecules that promote the growth of good bacteria, particularly Bifidobacteria.Galactooligosaccharides (GOS): Found in dairy products and certain legumes, GOS are composed of galactose molecules that encourage the growth of Bifidobacteria and Lactobacillus.Inulin: Chicory root, Jerusalem artichokes, and dandelion greens contain inulin, a type of fructan that promotes the growth of healthy bacteria and increases mineral absorption.Resistant Starch: Resistant starch is found in foods such as green bananas, cooked and cooled potatoes, and legumes. It resists digestion in the small intestine and ferments in the colon, boosting the growth of healthy bacteria.Pectins are soluble fibers found in apples, citrus fruits, and carrots that produce a gel-like substance in the gut to promote the growth of healthy bacteria and aid digestion.

2. Mechanism of Action:Selective Fermentation: Beneficial gut bacteria preferentially ferment prebiotics, producing short-chain fatty acids (SCFAs) such as acetate, propionate, and butyrate. SCFAs provide energy to colon cells, keep the gut barrier intact, and reduce inflammation.Beneficial Bacterial Stimulation:

Prebiotics promote the growth and activity of beneficial bacteria by acting as a food supply for them, hence increasing gut microbiome balance and variety.Immune Modulation: Prebiotics improve immune function by stimulating the growth of beneficial bacteria that interact with immune cells, increasing anti-inflammatory responses, and lowering the risk of infections and autoimmune illnesses.

3. Health Benefits of Prebiotics:Digestive Health: Prebiotics promote regular bowel movements, reduce constipation, and relieve the symptoms of digestive diseases such as IBS. They also increase the growth of beneficial bacteria, which lowers the risk of infection and improves overall gut health.Immune Function: Prebiotics boost general immune function by strengthening the gut barrier and modifying immunological responses, lowering the risk of infection and autoimmune illness.Metabolic Health: Prebiotics help regulate metabolism and body weight. They can boost insulin sensitivity, lower inflammation, and aid with weight management.Bone Health: Prebiotics increase mineral absorption, such as calcium and magnesium, which promotes bone health and lowers the risk of osteoporosis.Mental Health: The gut-brain axis links gut health and mental health. Prebiotics can improve mood and cognitive performance by lowering inflammation and promoting the growth of beneficial microorganisms.

Incorporating probiotics and prebiotics in your diet

Including probiotics and prebiotics in your diet is critical for maintaining a healthy gut microbiota. Here are some practical recommendations and tactics for incorporating these healthy components into your everyday meals:

1. Incorporating probiotics Yogurt: Select plain, unsweetened yogurt with live, active cultures. Add fresh fruits, nuts, or seeds to boost nutrition and flavor. Kefir: Kefir can be consumed as a drink or blended into smoothies for a probiotic boost. Choose basic, unsweetened types, and investigate dairy-free alternatives such as coconut or almond kefir. Sauerkraut and Kimchi: Use these fermented veggies in salads, sandwiches, or as a side dish. To preserve the probiotic content, make sure they're raw and unpasteurized. Miso: Add miso paste to soups, marinades, and sauces. Avoid boiling miso because high temperatures can kill the beneficial bacteria. Tempeh: Add tempeh to stir-fries, salads, and sandwiches. It is a diverse protein source and an excellent method to incorporate probiotics into your diet.Pickles: Choose organically fermented pickles without vinegar. Add them to sandwiches, salads, or eat them as a snack.

2. Incorporating prebioticsGarlic and Onions: Use garlic and onions as a base while cooking. They add flavor to recipes and include prebiotic fibers. Roast, sauté, or include them in soups and stews.Cook asparagus and artichokes by steaming, roasting, or grilling. They make great side dishes or complements to salads and noodles.Bananas: Eat them as a snack, in smoothies, or sliced over yogurt and porridge. They provide a convenient supply of prebiotics.Chicory Root: Chicory root can be used to replace coffee or added to smoothies and baked goods to provide a prebiotic boost.Whole Grains: Add whole grains like oats, quinoa, barley, and brown rice to your diet. They contain fiber and prebiotics, which promote intestinal health.Legumes: Add beans, lentils, and peas to your meals. They are high in prebiotic fiber and contain plant-based protein.

3. Combining probiotics and prebiotics: Make a probiotic smoothie by blending kefir or yogurt with prebiotic-rich foods such as bananas, berries, and a handful of spinach. For added fiber and omega-3s, mix in a teaspoon of flaxseeds or chia seeds.Prebiotic Salad: Start with leafy greens and then add sliced onions, garlic, asparagus, and artichokes. Add a spoonful of sauerkraut or kimchi for a probiotic boost.Fermented Food Bowls: Fill a bowl with various fermented foods, such as tempeh, miso, and kimchi. For a complete meal, combine prebiotic veggies such as roasted garlic and onions with healthy grains.Yogurt Parfait: Combine plain yogurt, sliced bananas, berries, and a sprinkle of oats or granola. Drizzle with honey for a natural sweetness.

4. Cooking Tips and Recipes:Probiotic-Rich Recipes.

Miso Soup: To make a simple miso soup, dissolve the miso paste in warm (but not boiling) water. For added nutrients, combine tofu, seaweed, and green onions.Fermented Veggies: To make your own fermented vegetables, combine shredded cabbage, carrots, and radishes with salt. Pack them into a jar and leave them to ferment at room temperature for a few days.Tempeh Stir-Fry: Sauté tempeh with your preferred vegetables and a splash of soy sauce or tamari. Serve with brown rice or quinoa.

Prebiotic-Rich Recipes:Roasted Garlic and Onion Soup: Roast garlic and onions until caramelized, then combine with vegetable broth and a splash of coconut milk to make a creamy soup.Banana Oat Pancakes: Combine mashed bananas, oats, eggs, and a touch of cinnamon. Serve with a dollop of yogurt and some fresh fruit.Chicory Root Coffee: Brew chicory root powder like coffee and drink it warm. If desired, serve with a splash of plant-based milk.

5. Supplements:Probiotic Supplements: If your diet does not provide enough probiotics, consider taking a supplement. Choose a high-quality product with a diverse range of strains and an adequate colony-forming unit (CFU) count. Consult with a healthcare expert to establish the best type and dose for your needs.Prebiotic Supplements: Inulin powder or GOS can be mixed into smoothies, baked goods, or beverages. They are an easy way to increase your consumption of prebiotics, especially if your dietary options are limited.

Chapter 5

Lifestyle Changes to Improve Digestion

The importance of hydration.

Hydration is crucial for sustaining good gut health. Water is important for all body functions, including digestion. Adequate hydration promotes the entire digestion process, from saliva production to nutrition absorption and waste removal. Understanding the importance of water and practicing good hydration habits can dramatically improve intestinal health.

1. The Role of Water in Digestion:Saliva Production: Digestion starts in the mouth, where saliva reacts with food to initiate the breakdown process. Saliva contains enzymes like amylase, which start the digestion of carbohydrates. Proper hydration promotes enough saliva production, which aids in the efficient breakdown of food.Mucus creation: Water promotes the creation of mucus in the digestive tract, which protects the stomach lining from acidic digestive fluids and allows food to flow smoothly through the intestines.Nutrient Absorption: Water dissolves nutrients and minerals, making them available for absorption in the intestine. Proper hydration is required for the absorption of water-soluble vitamins, minerals, and nutrients.Digestive Enzyme Function: Adequate hydration ensures that digestive enzymes are properly diluted, allowing for the breakdown of proteins, lipids, and carbs.Waste Elimination: Water is required for the production and movement of feces. It prevents constipation by making the feces soft and easy to pass. Proper hydration promotes regular bowel movements and efficient waste removal from the body.

2. Effects of Dehydration:Constipation: Constipation is one of the most obvious and acute side effects of dehydration. When the body does not have enough water, it absorbs more water from the colon, producing hard, dry stools that are difficult to pass.Slowed Digestion: Dehydration can slow down the digestive process, causing bloating, pain, and a sense of fullness.Acid Reflux: Poor hydration can diminish mucus production in the stomach, increasing the risk of acid reflux and discomfort.Nutrient shortages: Chronic dehydration can limit nutrient absorption, resulting in shortages that harm general health.Increased Toxin Load: Dehydration impairs the clearance of waste products and toxins, causing a buildup of toxic chemicals in the body and negatively impacting gut health.

3. Hydration strategies: Drink at least eight 8-ounce glasses of water every day (about 2 liters). Individual needs can vary depending on exercise level, climate, and overall health.Water-Rich Foods: Include water-rich foods in your diet, such as watermelon, strawberries, and oranges, as well as vegetables like cucumbers, lettuce, and celery. These foods promote overall hydration and provide critical nutrients.Hydration Timing: Drink your water throughout the day. Drinking a considerable amount of water at once might strain the digestive system. To stay hydrated, drink water on a consistent basis.Beverage Options: Although water is the best option for hydration, herbal teas and coconut water can also help with fluid intake. Avoid sugary drinks and excessive coffee, which can dehydrate the body.Hydration Cues: Be aware of indicators of dehydration, such as dry mouth, dark urine, lethargy, and headaches. Thirst is a late indicator of dehydration, so drink water frequently, even if you don't feel thirsty.

Exercise and gut health.

Regular physical activity is essential for general health, and the advantages extend to the digestive system. Exercise has a variety of effects on gut health, including increasing gut motility and promoting a healthy microbiota. Understanding the link between exercise and digestion might help you make more educated lifestyle choices that promote good digestive health.

1. Advantages of Exercise for Digestion:Increased Gut Motility: Physical activity stimulates the muscles of the digestive tract, promoting peristalsis—the rhythmic contractions that transport food through the intestines. This helps to reduce constipation and encourages regular bowel movements.Lower Risk of Digestive Diseases: Regular exercise has been associated with a lower risk of digestive diseases such as irritable bowel syndrome

(IBS), gastroesophageal reflux disease (GERD), and diverticular disease. Exercise helps regulate bowel function and reduce inflammation, which improves overall gut health.Increased microbiota diversity: Exercise fosters a diverse and balanced gut microbiota, which is essential for digestive health. A healthy microbiome promotes digestion, nutrition absorption, and immunological function.Stress Reduction: Exercise is an effective stress reliever. Stress can have a negative influence on gut health by worsening diseases like IBS and causing inflammation. Regular physical activity can help reduce these effects and enhance digestive health.Weight Management: Regular exercise can help you maintain a healthy weight and avoid obesity-related digestive problems, including acid reflux and fatty liver disease. Weight management promotes total metabolic health.

2. Types of Exercises Good for Digestion:Aerobic Exercise: Walking, jogging, swimming, and cycling all raise your heart rate and generate intestinal contractions, which promote gut motility and regular bowel movements.Strength Training: Weightlifting and bodyweight workouts help to improve muscular tone and metabolic health. Strong core muscles help improve posture and relieve pressure on the digestive organs.Yoga and stretching: These exercises can help relieve intestinal discomfort and promote calm. Twists and forward bends massage the stomach organs, which improve digestion and reduce bloating.Mind-Body Exercises: Practices such as Tai Chi and Pilates mix movement and awareness to reduce stress and improve digestive function. These exercises emphasize controlled motions and deep breathing, which might help to relax the digestive tract.

3. Incorporating Exercise into Your Routine:Start Slowly: If you're new to fitness, begin with low-intensity exercises like strolling or mild yoga. As you gain fitness, gradually increase the intensity and duration of your workouts.Consistency is essential. Aim for at least 150 minutes of moderate aerobic activity or 75 minutes of vigorous aerobic activity each week, as well as muscle-strengthening activities two or more days per week.Post-Meal Activity: Light exercise, such as a short stroll, can help digestion by increasing intestinal movement. Avoid intense exercise right after eating because it can induce discomfort and intestinal trouble.Hydration and Nutrition: Stay hydrated and eat nutritional foods to help your exercise regimen. Proper hydration is necessary for peak performance and digestion.Listen to Your Body: Pay attention to how your body reacts to various forms of exercise. If you feel gastric discomfort while or after exercising, modify the intensity, duration, or kind of activity.

Sleep and its impact on digestion.

Sleep is an essential component of good health that has a significant impact on digestive function. Sleep and digestion have a bidirectional relationship: poor sleep can have a detrimental impact on gut health, and digestive disorders can disrupt sleep. Understanding this association and implementing appropriate sleep habits can help improve both sleep quality and intestinal health.

1. The Gut and Sleep Connection:Circadian Rhythms: The digestive system follows a circadian rhythm, which governs the timing of digestive functions such as enzyme production, gut motility, and nutrient absorption. Disrupted sleep habits can upset these rhythms, resulting in digestive problems.Gut Microbiome: The gut microbiome likewise has a circadian rhythm, with specific bacterial activities peaking at different times of day. Poor sleep can change the composition and function of the gut microbiome, leading to digestive issues.Hormonal Regulation: Sleep influences the production of hormones including ghrelin and leptin, which govern hunger, fullness, and digestion. Disrupted sleep can cause hormone imbalances, increased hunger, and altered intestinal function.Inflammation: Poor sleep quality and sleep loss can cause inflammation throughout the body, including the stomach. Chronic inflammation can worsen digestive issues and harm gut health.

2. Poor sleep can have a negative impact on digestion.Increased Gastrointestinal Symptoms: Inadequate sleep is linked to an increase in gastrointestinal symptoms such as bloating, constipation, diarrhea, and stomach pain.Exacerbation of Digestive Disorders: Conditions such as IBS, GERD, and inflammatory bowel disease (IBD) might worsen due to poor sleep quality. Sleep problems can cause flare-ups and worsen symptoms.Changed Gut Motility: Disrupted sleep patterns can impair gut motility, resulting in irregular bowel motions and disorders such as constipation or diarrhea.Weight Gain: Inadequate sleep can cause weight gain by increasing appetite and affecting metabolism. Excess weight can lead to digestive problems such as acid reflux and fatty liver disease.

3. Strategies to Improve Sleep and Digestion:Create a Sleep Routine: Maintain a consistent sleep schedule by going to bed and waking up at the same time every day, including weekends. This helps to manage your body's circadian rhythm.Create a Sleep-Friendly Environment: Keep your bedroom cold, dark, and quiet. Use comfy beds and keep noise and light out.Limit stimulants: Avoid caffeine and nicotine close to bedtime, as these might disrupt sleep. Also, minimize your alcohol consumption because it can interfere with your sleep.Healthy Eating Habits: Avoid heavy, fatty, or spicy meals before bedtime since they can induce intestinal pain and interfere with sleep. If you need to eat something before bed, choose light, easily digestible nibbles.Relaxation Techniques: Practice relaxation techniques like deep breathing, meditation, or moderate yoga.

Before going to bed, minimize tension and promote better sleep.Physical Activity: Regular exercise can enhance sleep quality, but avoid strenuous exercise close to bedtime because it can be stimulating and disrupt sleep.Limit Screen Time: Limit your exposure to screens (phones, laptops, and televisions) at least an hour before bedtime. Screens emit blue light, which can interfere with melatonin production and interrupt sleep.Hydration Balance: Stay hydrated throughout the day, but restrict fluid intake before bedtime to avoid waking up at night to use the bathroom.

Chapter 6

Heal and Restore Your Gut

Identifying Food Sensitivity and Allergies

Food sensitivities and allergies can have a substantial impact on gut health, resulting in inflammation, discomfort, and a variety of digestive disorders. Identifying and managing these disorders is critical to your gut's repair and restoration. Understanding the distinction between food sensitivities and allergies, detecting symptoms, and using identification tactics are all critical aspects of this process.

1. Understanding Food Sensitivity and Allergy:Food Allergies: A food allergy is an immune system reaction to a specific dietary protein. This reaction can be severe, even life-threatening. Common food allergens include peanuts, tree nuts, shellfish, fish, milk, eggs, soy, and wheat. Symptoms range from hives, edema, and stomach problems to anaphylaxis.Food Sensitivity: Unlike allergies, food sensitivities (or intolerances) do not affect the immune system. They happen when the digestive system has trouble processing particular foods. Lactose, gluten, and certain food additives are among the most common causes. Bloating, gas, diarrhea, and abdominal pain are common symptoms, but they are usually mild.

2. Recognizing symptoms:Digestive Symptoms: Bloating, gas, diarrhea, constipation, and stomach discomfort are frequent signs of food sensitivities and allergies.Skin Reactions: Eczema, hives, and other skin irritations may suggest a food allergy or sensitivities.Respiratory Symptoms: Food allergies are associated with wheezing, coughing, and nasal congestion, but sensitivities can also cause these symptoms.Systemic Reactions: Food sensitivities can cause fatigue, headaches, and joint discomfort, which are symptoms of systemic inflammation.Neurological symptoms: Food sensitivities can cause brain fog, mood swings, and anxiety, emphasizing the gut-brain connection.

3. Strategies for identification:Elimination Diet: This entails removing suspicious foods from your diet for a period of time (usually 2-4 weeks) before gradually returning them one at a time. Monitoring symptoms during reintroduction can assist in identifying triggers.Food journal: Keeping a detailed food journal might aid in tracking what you eat and any symptoms that arise. This can provide useful insights and aid in identifying patterns.Allergy Testing: Skin prick tests and blood testing (such as the ImmunoCAP test) can be used to diagnose particular food allergies. These tests should be carried out under the supervision of a healthcare practitioner.Sensitivity Testing: Although there are several tests available for food sensitivities (such as IgG antibody tests), their reliability is questioned. An elimination diet is still the gold standard for discovering sensitivities.

Detoxify your gut

Detoxification entails eliminating toxic compounds from the body while assisting the liver and kidneys in their natural detoxification activities. A gut detox aims to eliminate toxins, reduce inflammation, and improve gut health through dietary and lifestyle modifications.

1. Removing ToxinsAvoid processed meals: processed meals frequently contain additives, preservatives, and artificial components, which can harm gut health. Concentrate on whole, natural foods.Limit Sugar Intake: Excess sugar can encourage the growth of pathogenic bacteria and yeast, resulting in dysbiosis. Reduce your consumption of sugary meals and beverages.Limit alcohol and caffeine. Both can irritate the stomach lining and upset the balance of the gut flora. Moderation is crucial.Avoid Artificial Sweeteners: Certain artificial sweeteners can harm the gut microbiota. Use natural sweeteners like honey or maple syrup in tiny amounts.

2. Supporting the liver:Cruciferous Vegetables: Broccoli, Brussels sprouts, and Kale contain chemicals that help the liver detoxify.Antioxidant-rich foods:

Berries, citrus fruits, nuts, and seeds contain antioxidants that help protect the liver from oxidative stress.Hydration: Drinking plenty of water helps the kidneys operate and clear away toxins.

3. Promoting gut health:Fiber-Rich Foods: Fiber promotes regular bowel movements and aids in the removal of waste and toxins from the body. Include a variety of fruits, vegetables, whole grains, and legumes.Fermented foods contain helpful microorganisms that promote a healthy gut microbiota. Add yogurt, kefir, sauerkraut, and kimchi to your diet.Prebiotic Foods: Foods such as garlic, onions, asparagus, and bananas nourish good bacteria, promoting gut health and detox.Probiotics: Consider taking a high-quality probiotic supplement to help restore healthy microorganisms.

4. Detoxing Practices:Intermittent fasting: This allows your digestive system to rest and supports natural cleansing processes.Herbal teas, such as dandelion, ginger, and peppermint, can aid digestion and cleansing.Exercise: Regular physical activity improves circulation and aids in the removal of pollutants via perspiration.Stress Management: Yoga, meditation, and deep breathing exercises can help reduce stress and improve gut health.

Natural remedies and supplements.

Natural therapies and supplements can help to repair and restore gut health. They can help reduce inflammation, improve digestion, and restore good bacteria. Here are some useful natural therapies and supplements for gut health:

1. Herbal remedies:Ginger: Ginger is known for its anti-inflammatory and digestive characteristics, which can help reduce nausea, promote digestion, and relieve bloating. It can be enjoyed as tea or mixed into meals.Peppermint: Peppermint oil contains antispasmodic qualities that can help with IBS symptoms like stomach pain and bloating. Peppermint tea is very comforting to the digestive system.Turmeric contains curcumin, a potent anti-inflammatory substance that promotes intestinal health. Incorporate turmeric into your diet by cooking it or taking it as a supplement.Slippery Elm: When combined with water, this herb produces a calming gel that can protect the gut lining and relieve inflammation. It is commonly used to treat the symptoms of IBS and IBD.

2. Digestive enzymes:Supplementing with Enzymes: Digestive enzymes can aid in the breakdown of meals and boost nutritional absorption. They are especially beneficial for people who have enzyme deficits or are experiencing bloating and indigestion.Sources: Enzyme supplements frequently comprise protease, lipase, amylase, and lactase. They can be taken before a meal to help digestion.

3. Probiotics:Supplementing with Probiotics: Probiotic supplements can help replenish beneficial bacteria and restore gut microbiome equilibrium. Look for a high-quality supplement with a variety of strains and an adequate CFU count.Specific Strains: Each probiotic strain provides unique benefits. Lactobacillus rhamnosus GG, for example, helps treat diarrhea, while Bifidobacterium longum can alleviate IBS symptoms.

4. Prebiotics:Prebiotic Supplements: When food sources are limited, prebiotic supplements can promote the growth of beneficial microorganisms. Common prebiotic supplements include inulin and fructooligosaccharides (FOS).Combination Products: Some supplements combine probiotics and prebiotics (synbiotics) to increase the synergistic effects.

5.Omega-3 Fatty Acids:Anti-Inflammatory Benefits: Omega-3 fatty acids have strong anti-inflammatory qualities that promote intestinal health. They can help reduce inflammation in disorders like IBD and promote overall digestive health.Sources: Consume fatty fish (such as salmon, mackerel, and sardines), flaxseeds, chia seeds, and walnuts in your diet. Omega-3 supplements, such as fish oil and algal oil, are also available.

6. Glutamine:Gut Repair: Glutamine is an amino acid that helps to repair and regenerate the gut lining. It is especially useful for people who have leaky gut syndrome, or IBD.Supplementation: Glutamine supplements can be used to help the gut repair itself. It is frequently advised to consume it on an empty stomach for maximum absorption.

7. Aloe vera:Soothing Effects: Aloe vera's soothing and anti-inflammatory properties can aid in the healing of the stomach lining and the reduction of IBS and acid reflux symptoms.Consumption: Aloe vera juice should be drunk in moderation to promote intestinal health. Make sure it is free of aloin, a chemical that might cause laxative effects.

8. Apple Cider Vinegar:Digestive Aid: Apple cider vinegar stimulates stomach acid production and improves digestion. It may help relieve the symptoms of indigestion and acid reflux.Directions: Dilute a spoonful of apple cider vinegar in a glass of water and consume before meals. If you have a sensitive stomach or have acid reflux, proceed with caution.

9. Bone broth:Nutrient-dense: Bone broth contains collagen, gelatin, and amino acids such as glutamine, which aid in gut healing and repair. It also offers the necessary minerals.To make bone broth, boil bones with water, veggies, and seasonings for many hours. It can be drunk warm or used as a soup or stew foundation.

10.Fiber Supplements:Supporting Regularity: Fiber supplements such as psyllium husk can help with regular bowel movements and overall gut health. They add weight to the feces and encourage the growth of good bacteria.Types: Soluble fiber supplements dissolve in water to form a gel-like substance, whereas insoluble fiber adds bulk to the stool. Choose a supplement that meets your individual needs.

Chapter 7

The Mind-Gut Connection.

How Stress Impacts Your Gut

The mind and gut are linked by a complex network of neurological, hormonal, and immunological processes. This relationship, known as the "gut-brain axis," emphasizes the powerful influence that mental and emotional states, particularly stress, can have on digestive health. Understanding how stress affects the stomach is critical for treating digestive issues and improving overall health.

1. The Gut-Brain Axis:Bidirectional Communication: The gut-brain axis allows for bidirectional communication between the central nervous system (CNS) and the enteric nervous system (ENS). The ENS, sometimes known as the "second brain," controls gastrointestinal function and communicates with the CNS via the vagus nerve, neurotransmitters, and hormones.Neurotransmitters: Neurotransmitters such as serotonin and dopamine play important roles in mood regulation and gastrointestinal function. Interestingly, the gut contains around 95% of the body's serotonin, which influences gut motility, secretion, and feeling.Hormonal Influence: Stress causes the release of stress hormones, including cortisol and adrenaline, which can impair gut motility, permeability, and inflammation. These hormones prepare the body for a "fight or flight" reaction, but their prolonged activation might impair digestive processes.

2. Physiological Effects of Stress on the Gut:Changed Gut Motility: Stress can cause either increased or decreased gut motility. Acute stress can cause diarrhea owing to the short transit time, whereas persistent stress can decrease motility, resulting in constipation.Gut

Permeability: Stress can increase gut permeability, often known as "leaky gut." This allows hazardous chemicals such as toxins and bacteria to flow through the stomach lining into the circulation, prompting an immunological response and inflammation.Microbiome Imbalance: Chronic stress can upset the equilibrium of the gut microbiota, lowering the diversity and number of beneficial bacteria. This dysbiosis can lead to stomach problems, inflammation, and a compromised immune system.Inflammation: Stress-related inflammation can aggravate illnesses such as irritable bowel syndrome (IBS) and inflammatory bowel disease (IBD). Pro-inflammatory cytokines produced in reaction to stress can exacerbate gut inflammation and symptoms.

3.Emotional and behavioral effects:Increased Sensitivity: Stress can increase the gut's sensitivity, making people more vulnerable to pain and discomfort. Increased visceral sensitivity is a typical trait in disorders such as IBS.Changes in Eating Habits: Stress can cause changes in appetite and eating behavior, such as bingeing, undereating, or seeking harmful foods. These dietary modifications may have a further impact on gut health.Sleep Disruption: Stress frequently interrupts sleep, and poor sleep quality can harm gut health, creating a vicious cycle.

Mindfulness and meditation for gut health.

Mindfulness and meditation techniques have acquired global recognition for their capacity to reduce stress, improve emotional control, and boost general well-being. These techniques can help improve gut health by regulating the gut-brain axis and encouraging a balanced, healthy digestive system.

1. **Mindfulness and its Benefits:Definition:** Mindfulness is the practice of paying attention to the present moment without judgment. It promotes awareness of thoughts,feelings, physiological sensations, and surroundings.Stress Reduction: Mindfulness techniques help people relax and respond to stressors in a more balanced way. This can help relieve stress-related gastrointestinal symptoms and enhance digestive function.Improved Gut-Brain Communication: By cultivating a conscious awareness of physical sensations, people can better tune in to their gut's messages and respond accordingly, potentially lowering the symptoms of digestive diseases.

2. **Meditation and its Benefits:Meditation Types:** Mindfulness meditation, guided meditation, and loving-kindness meditation are all beneficial to gut health. These activities include focusing attention,

creating pleasant emotions, and achieving inner calm.Neural Changes: Meditation has been found to improve brain structure and function, particularly in regions responsible for emotional control, attention, and self-awareness. These adjustments can boost stress resilience and intestinal health.Hormonal Regulation: Meditation helps reduce stress chemicals such as cortisol, which have a harmful impact on the gut. It can also stimulate the release of feel-good neurotransmitters such as serotonin, which improves mood and gastrointestinal function.

3. Practical Mindfulness and Meditation Techniques:Mindful Eating: This technique entails paying close attention to the eating experience, including the taste, texture, and smell of food, as well as the body's hunger and satiety cues. Mindful eating can improve digestion, prevent overeating, and increase enjoyment of food.Breath Awareness: Concentrating on your breath is a basic yet effective mindfulness technique. It entails focusing on the natural rhythm of breathing, which can improve relaxation and alleviate stress-related gastrointestinal symptoms.Body Scan Meditation: In this technique, you mentally scan your entire body from head to toe, detecting any feelings without judgment. It can help people become more conscious of their gut feelings and respond to discomfort more calmly.Guided Imagery: Guided imagery entails visualizing tranquil and relaxing images or events. This activity can lower stress, induce relaxation, and improve gut health.Loving-Kindness Meditation: This type of meditation aims to cultivate feelings of compassion and love for oneself and others. It can relieve stress and improve mental well-being, hence indirectly boosting intestinal health.

Strategies for managing stress

Effective stress management is vital for gut health and general well-being. Several measures can help reduce stress, improve emotional regulation, and promote digestive health. Here are some evidence-based ways to manage stress:

1.Lifestyle modifications:Regular Exercise: Physical activity is an effective stress reducer. Exercise produces endorphins, which boost mood and induce relaxation. Aim for at least 150 minutes of moderate aerobic activity or 75 minutes of strenuous activity per week, with strength training activities.Balanced Diet: Eating a nutritious diet promotes general health and resilience to stress. Concentrate on whole foods, including fruits, vegetables, lean meats, whole grains, and healthy fats. Avoid excessive caffeine, sugar, and processed foods, which can aggravate stress.Adequate Sleep: Prioritize proper sleep hygiene to ensure comfortable, rejuvenating sleep. Maintain a consistent sleep schedule, create a relaxing sleeping environment, and limit screen time before bedtime. Aim for 7-9 hours of sleep each night.

2. Relaxation techniques:Deep Breathing: Deep, diaphragmatic breathing activates the parasympathetic nervous system, which promotes relaxation and reduces stress. Try the 4-7-8 breathing technique or box breathing.Progressive Muscle Calm: This technique involves tensing and then relaxing various muscle groups, which promotes both physical and mental calm. It can help reduce stress and enhance sleep quality.Aromatherapy: Using essential oils such as lavender, chamomile, and eucalyptus can help you relax and relieve tension. Aromatherapy can be incorporated into a variety of techniques, including diffusing oils, adding them to baths, and lighting scented candles.

3. Cognitive and behavioral approaches:Cognitive-BBehavioral Therapy (CBT): CBT is a well-known therapy method for identifying and changing negative thought patterns and behaviors. It is effective at reducing stress, anxiety, and depression, which can improve gut health.Stress Journaling: Keeping a journal to record stressors and emotional responses might help people understand their stress patterns and build coping methods. Writing about stress might also help you feel better and process your emotions.Time Management: Effective time management can reduce stress by assisting individuals in prioritizing activities, setting realistic goals, and avoiding procrastination. To-do lists, deadlines, and breaking down activities into manageable parts are all effective techniques.

4. Social and emotional support:Social Connections: Establishing and maintaining strong social connections can help with emotional support and stress reduction. Spend time with your family and friends, join social clubs, and participate in community events.Communication Skills: Learning excellent communication skills can help people express their needs, create boundaries, and settle disagreements, lowering stress in interpersonal relationships.Therapeutic Support: Seeking help from a therapist or counselor can provide a secure environment in which to discuss stressors, learn coping techniques, and receive emotional support. Therapy can be especially effective for dealing with persistent stress and emotional issues.

5. Mind/Body Practices:Yoga: Yoga combines physical postures, breath control, and meditation to help you relax and reduce stress. It can boost flexibility, strength, and mental clarity, promoting general well-being and intestinal health.Tai Chi and Qigong: These ancient Chinese techniques consist of slow, deliberate motions, deep breathing, and concentration. They encourage relaxation, balance, and stress reduction, which improve both mental and physical health.Mindfulness-Based

Stress Reduction (MBSR): MBSR is an evidence-based approach that uses mindfulness meditation and yoga to reduce stress and promote overall well-being. It has been demonstrated to improve symptoms of anxiety, sadness, and chronic pain.

6. Creative Outlets: Art and Music Therapy: Creative activities such as drawing, painting, playing an instrument, or listening to music can help with emotional expression and stress reduction. Art and music therapy can help people relax and enhance their mood.Hobbies and Interests: Pursuing hobbies and interests that bring you joy and fulfillment can be a good way to de-stress and feel accomplished. Activities such as gardening, cooking, reading, and crafting might be useful.

Chapter 8

Personalized Gut Health Plans.

Creating a Gut Health Journal

Keeping a gut health journal is a useful and effective way to monitor and improve your digestive health. By documenting various parts of your nutrition, lifestyle, and symptoms, you can get insight into what impacts your gut and make more informed decisions to encourage better digestion and general well-being. Here's how to make and use a gut health journal effectively:

1. Setting up your journal:Format: Select a format that best meets your needs—it could be a real notepad, a digital document, or a customized app. The trick is to choose a method that you will regularly use.Sections: Divide your journal into sections to monitor various aspects of your gut health. Sections to consider include daily food intake, symptoms, bowel motions, water, physical activity, stress levels, sleep quality, and supplements or medications.

2. Daily Food Intake:Detailed logging: Keep track of everything you eat and drink throughout the day. Include the time of intake, amount quantities, and any specifics (for example, how the dish was made and what ingredients were used).Food Categories: Keep track of the things you consume, such as fruits, vegetables, proteins, grains, dairy, fermented foods, processed foods, and so on. This can help uncover trends associated with various meal categories.

3. Symptoms:Symptom Logging: Record any digestive symptoms you have, such as bloating, gas, constipation, diarrhea, heartburn, nausea, or abdominal discomfort. Note the degree and duration of each symptom. Timing and Triggers: Keep track of when symptoms arise in connection with meals, stressors, physical activity, or other possible triggers. This can aid in detecting relationships and determining specific causes.

4. Bowel Movements:Frequency and Consistency: Using a scale like the Bristol Stool Chart, keep track of how frequently and consistently your bowel motions occur. This can aid in detecting patterns and potential problems, such as constipation or diarrhea.Other features: Take note of any extra features, such as color, odor, and the presence of blood or mucus, as these can provide valuable information about your digestive health.

5. Hydration:Fluid Intake: Keep track of how much water and other liquids you consume each day. Keep track of the amount and type of fluids consumed.Hydration Status: Keep track of indicators of dehydration, such as dark urine, dry mouth, or weariness, and write them in your journal.

6. Physical Activity:Exercise Log: Keep track of your daily physical activity, including the type, duration, and intensity of the exercise. This might help you determine the effect of physical activity on your digestive health.Post-Exercise Observations: Take note of any digestive changes or symptoms that appear after exercise, such as improved bowel movements or discomfort.

7. Stress levels:Stress Tracking: Keep track of your daily stress levels, including any major stressors or events. To quantify your stress level, use a scale (such as 1–10).Coping Mechanisms: Keep track of any stress management techniques you use, such as meditation, deep breathing, or leisure activities, and how effective they are in relieving stress.

8. Sleep Quality:Sleep Patterns: Keep track of your sleep length and quality every night. Take note of the times you go to bed and wake up, as well as any interruptions or difficulty falling asleep.Sleep Impact: Observe and document any links between sleep quality and digestive problems. Poor sleep can exacerbate digestive troubles, but adequate sleep can improve digestion.

9. Supplements and medications:Supplement Log: Keep track of any supplements or drugs you take, including their dosage and time. This can help uncover potential interactions or side effects.Observations: Take note of any changes in symptoms or overall well-being as a result of supplement or medicine use.

Tailoring your diet and lifestyle

Understanding your own needs, preferences, and reactions to various foods and activities is necessary when personalizing your diet and lifestyle to support gut health. Analyzing data from your gut health journal allows you to detect patterns and make focused changes to improve your digestive health.

1. Analyzing Journal Data:Pattern Recognition: Examine your diary entries for patterns or relationships between food intake, symptoms, and other variables. Look for trends, such as certain foods causing persistent discomfort or specific activities that improve digestion.Trigger Identification: Determine any probable food or lifestyle triggers that may be contributing to your digestive problems. Common triggers include dairy, gluten, high-fat diets, spicy foods, and stress.

2. Elimination and Reintroduction:Elimination Phase: If you feel that certain foods are producing symptoms, consider an elimination diet by excluding certain foods from your diet for a set length of time (usually 2-4 weeks). Dairy, gluten, soy, and high-FODMAP foods are common things to remove.Reintroduction Phase: Gradually reintroduce removed foods one at a time, observing your body's reaction. This can aid in determining specific dietary sensitivities or intolerances.

3. Dietary adjustments:Increase Fiber Intake: Make sure your diet contains enough fiber-rich foods such as fruits, vegetables, whole grains, legumes, nuts, and seeds. Fiber promotes normal bowel movements and a healthy gut microbiota.Incorporate Fermented Foods: Include fermented foods such as yogurt, kefir, sauerkraut, kimchi, and kombucha in your diet. These foods contain probiotics that promote intestinal health.Choose entire meals: opt for entire, minimally processed meals. Avoid processed foods heavy in sugar, bad fats, and artificial additives, as these might have a negative impact on gut health.Maintain a balanced macronutrient intake, including proteins, carbs, and fats. Each contributes significantly to general health and digestive function.Hydration: Stay properly hydrated by consuming plenty of water throughout the day. Proper water promotes digestion and prevents constipation.

4. Lifestyle adjustments:Stress Management: Try stress-reduction practices like mindfulness meditation, yoga, deep breathing exercises, or activities that you enjoy. Stress reduction can have a substantial positive impact on digestive health.Regular Exercise: Engage in enjoyable physical activity on a regular basis. Aim for a combination of cardio, strength, and flexibility exercises, such as yoga or stretching.Prioritize appropriate sleep hygiene routines to support peaceful, rejuvenating sleep. This involves adhering to a consistent sleep schedule, providing a relaxing sleep environment, and limiting screen time before bed.Mindful Eating: Pay attention to your food, chew carefully, and enjoy every bite. This can help you digest food better and avoid overeating.

5. Consulting with professionals: Consult a trained dietitian or nutritionist to create a personalized food plan based on your journal data and specific needs.Gastroenterologist: If you have persistent or severe digestive problems, consult a gastroenterologist. They can offer specialist testing and treatment options for IBS, IBD, and food intolerances.Mental health expert: If stress, anxiety, or other mental health concerns have a substantial impact on your digestive health, you should get help from a mental health expert. Cognitive-behavioral therapy (CBT) can help manage stress and its effects on the stomach.

Long-term Strategies to Maintain Gut Health

Maintaining gut health is a lifelong adventure that requires constant monitoring and adjustment to your diet, lifestyle, and overall well-being. Long-term tactics can help maintain gut health and prevent prospective problems.

1. Ongoing monitoring and adjustments:Continued Journaling: Keep your gut health journal to track ongoing trends and find new triggers or patterns. This can help you be more proactive in controlling your digestive health.Seasonal Adjustments: Change your diet and lifestyle to reflect seasonal variations. For example, in the summer, include more hydrating foods and lighter meals, while in the winter, emphasize warming, nutrient-dense foods.Routine Check-Ins: Review your journal and overall health on a regular basis. Make the required changes to your nutrition, exercise routine, stress management strategies, and sleeping habits.

2. Supporting Gut Microbiome Diversity:Dietary Variety: Eat a variety of foods to maintain a healthy and diverse gut microbiota. Different meals include different minerals and fibers, which nourish various beneficial microorganisms.Prebiotic Foods: Consume prebiotic-rich foods such as garlic, onions, leeks, asparagus, bananas, and whole grains. Prebiotics are nondigestible fibers that nourish healthy intestinal microorganisms.Probiotic Supplements: Take a high-quality probiotic supplement, especially if you've recently taken antibiotics or had digestive issues. Probiotics can help restore and maintain a healthy balance of gut bacteria.

3. Mindfulness Eating Practices:Chewing your food completely: Chew your food completely to help digestion and nutritional absorption. Chewing also stimulates the body to manufacture digestive enzymes.Eating Regularly: Stick to regular meal times and avoid skipping meals. Consistent eating patterns promote steady blood sugar levels and proper digestive function.Listen to Your Body: Pay attention to your body's hunger and fullness signals. Eat when you're hungry and stop when you're full, rather than eating for habit or boredom.

4. Managing stress:Consistent Practices: Use stress management approaches that are effective for you on a regular basis. Consistency is essential for lowering the overall effect of stress on your gut health.Work/Life Balance

Strive for a healthy work-life balance. Make time for leisure, hobbies, and social activities that are enjoyable and stress-reducing.Support Systems: Rely on family, friends, and support groups. Sharing your experiences and receiving support can greatly relieve stress.

5. Physical Activity:Exercise: Maintain a consistent exercise regimen that includes a variety of aerobic, strength, and flexibility exercises. Aim to do at least 150 minutes of moderate exercise per week.Active Lifestyle: Include physical activities in your regular routine. Simple modifications, such as using the stairs, walking or biking instead of driving, and participating in active activities, can help improve overall health.

6. Quality sleep:Sleep Routine: Follow a consistent sleep schedule, especially on weekends. Consistency regulates your body's internal schedule and promotes sleep quality.Sleep Environment: Keep your bedroom cold, dark, and quiet to promote restful sleep. Consider wearing earplugs or an eye mask, if necessary.Relaxation Techniques: Before going to bed, try relaxing activities like reading, having a warm bath, or listening to soothing music. Avoid engaging in stimulating activities such as watching television or using electronic devices.

7. Regular health checkups:Medical Checkups: Make regular appointments with your healthcare practitioner to examine your overall health and treat any growing difficulties. Routine screenings and tests can assist in detecting problems early.Lab testing: Consider getting periodic lab testing to evaluate gut health markers like inflammation, vitamin deficits, and microbial diversity. Your healthcare practitioner can recommend tests that are appropriate for your requirements.

8. Education and awareness:Stay Informed: Keep up with the most recent gut health research and information. Understanding new discoveries might help you make more informed choices about your food and lifestyle.Educational Resources: To learn more about gut health, read books, articles, podcasts, and visit credible websites. Educating oneself allows you to be proactive in maintaining your digestive health.

Chapter 9

Recipes for Gut Health

Breakfasts: Starting Your Day Right

A nutritious and balanced breakfast sets the tone for the rest of the day. A gut-friendly breakfast includes fiber, protein, healthy fats, and probiotics to promote optimal digestion and sustained energy. Here are some delicious recipes to start your day right.

1. Gut-Healing Smoothie Bowl

Ingredients:

1 cup unsweetened almond milk or coconut milk

1 frozen banana

1/2 cup frozen berries (blueberries, strawberries, or raspberries)

1/4 cup plain Greek yogurt (for probiotics)

1 tablespoon chia seeds (for fiber)

1 tablespoon of flaxseeds (for omega-3 fatty acids)

1 tablespoon almond butter (for healthy fats)

1 handful of spinach or kale (for fiber and vitamins)

Toppings:

Fresh berries

Sliced banana

Granola (preferably homemade or low-sugar)

Coconut flakes

Instructions:

1. In a blender, combine the almond milk, frozen banana, frozen berries, Greek yogurt, chia seeds, flaxseeds, almond butter, and spinach or kale.

2. Blend until smooth and creamy.

3. Pour the smoothie into a bowl and top with fresh berries, sliced banana, granola, and coconut flakes.

4. Enjoy immediately as a nutritious and filling breakfast.

2. Overnight Oats with Chia Seeds

Ingredients:

1/2 cup rolled oats

1 cup unsweetened almond milk or coconut milk

2 tablespoons of chia seeds

1/2 teaspoon vanilla extract

1 tablespoon honey or maple syrup (optional)

1/4 cup mixed berries (fresh or frozen)

1/4 cup chopped nuts (almonds, walnuts, or pecans)

Instructions:

1. In a mason jar or bowl, combine the rolled oats, almond milk, chia seeds, vanilla extract, and honey or maple syrup (if using).

2. Stir well to combine and ensure the chia seeds are evenly distributed.

3. Cover and refrigerate overnight or for at least 4 hours.

4. In the morning, stir the oats again and top with mixed berries and chopped nuts.

5. Enjoy a delicious and fiber-rich breakfast that promotes good gut health.

3. Probiotic-rich Greek Yogurt Parfait

Ingredients:

1 cup of plain Greek yogurt

1/2 cup granola (preferably homemade or low-sugar)

1/2 cup mixed berries (blueberries, strawberries, or raspberries)

1 tablespoon of honey or maple syrup

1 tablespoon of chia seeds

1 tablespoon pumpkin seeds (for added crunch)

Instructions:

1. In a glass or bowl, layer half of the Greek yogurt.

2. Add a layer of granola and a layer of mixed berries.

3. Repeat the layers with the remaining yogurt, granola, and berries.

4. Drizzle honey or maple syrup over the top and sprinkle with chia seeds and pumpkin seeds.

5. Enjoy a delicious and probiotic-rich breakfast that supports gut health.

4. Avocado Toast with Fermented Veggies

Ingredients:

1 slice of whole-grain or sourdough bread

1 ripe avocado

1/4 cup fermented vegetables (such as sauerkraut or kimchi)

1 tablespoon of hemp seeds (for added nutrients)

Salt and pepper to taste

Optional: red pepper flakes for a bit of spice.

Instructions:

1. Toast the slice of whole-grain or sourdough bread to your liking.

2. While the bread is toasting, mash the avocado in a bowl until smooth.

3. Spread the mashed avocado evenly over the toasted bread.

4. Top with fermented vegetables and sprinkle with hemp seeds, salt, pepper, and red pepper flakes if desired.

5. Enjoy a gut-friendly breakfast that is rich in fiber, healthy fats, and probiotics.

Lunches: Midday Gut Boosters

A balanced lunch helps maintain energy levels and supports digestive health throughout the day. These recipes include plenty of fiber, lean protein, and gut-friendly ingredients to keep your digestive system running smoothly.

1. Quinoa and Black Bean Salad

Ingredients:

1 cup cooked quinoa

1 cup black beans, rinsed and drained

1/2 cup cherry tomatoes, halved

1/2 cup cucumber, diced

1/4 cup red onion, finely chopped

1/4 cup fresh cilantro, chopped

1 avocado, diced

Juice of 1 lime

2 tablespoons of olive oil

Salt and pepper to taste

Instructions:

1. In a large bowl, combine the cooked quinoa, black beans, cherry tomatoes, cucumber, red onion, and cilantro.

2. Add the diced avocado and gently mix to combine.

3. In a small bowl, whisk together the lime juice, olive oil, salt, and pepper.

4. Pour the dressing over the salad and toss to coat evenly.

5. Serve immediately or refrigerate for a few hours to let the flavors meld together. Enjoy a fiber-rich and protein-packed lunch.

2. Gut-Friendly Buddha Bowl

Ingredients:

1 cup cooked brown rice or quinoa

1 cup roasted or steamed vegetables (such as broccoli, sweet potatoes, or bell peppers)

1/2 cup chickpeas, rinsed and drained

1/4 cup sauerkraut or kimchi

1 avocado, sliced

1 tablespoon tahini

1 tablespoon of lemon juice

1 tablespoon of water

Salt and pepper to taste

Optional: sesame seeds or hemp seeds for garnish.

Instructions:

1. In a bowl, layer the cooked brown rice or quinoa as the base.

2. Arrange the roasted or steamed vegetables, chickpeas, sauerkraut or kimchi, and avocado slices on top.

3. In a small bowl, whisk together the tahini, lemon juice, water, salt, and pepper to create a creamy dressing.

4. Drizzle the dressing over the Buddha bowl and sprinkle with sesame seeds or hemp seeds if desired.

5. Enjoy a nutritious and gut-friendly lunch that is packed with fiber, protein, and probiotics.

3. Mediterranean Chickpea Wrap

Ingredients:

1 whole-grain or gluten-free wrap

1/2 cup chickpeas, rinsed and mashed

1/4 cup hummus

1/2 cup spinach or mixed greens

1/4 cup cucumber, thinly sliced

1/4 cup cherry tomatoes, halved

1/4 cup red onion, thinly sliced

2 tablespoons crumbled feta cheese (optional)

1 tablespoon of olive oil

Juice of 1/2 lemon

Salt and pepper to taste

Instructions:

1. In a small bowl, combine the mashed chickpeas, olive oil, lemon juice, salt, and pepper.

2. Spread the hummus evenly over the whole-grain wrap.

3. Layer the spinach or mixed greens, cucumber, cherry tomatoes, red onion, and crumbled feta cheese (if using) on top of the hummus.

4. Add the chickpea mixture and roll up the wrap tightly.

5. Slice in half and enjoy a delicious and fiber-rich lunch that supports gut health.

Dinners: Evening Digestive Support

A balanced and nutritious dinner can aid digestion and help you wind down after a long day. These recipes focus on lean proteins, vegetables, and gut-friendly ingredients to provide evening digestive support.

1. Baked Salmon with Asparagus and Quinoa

Ingredients:

2 salmon fillets

1 bunch of asparagus, trimmed

1 cup cooked quinoa

2 tablespoons of olive oil

1 lemon, sliced

2 cloves garlic, minced

Salt and pepper to taste

Fresh dill or parsley for garnish

Instructions:

1. Preheat the oven to 375°F (190°C).

2. Place the salmon fillets and asparagus on a baking sheet lined with parchment paper.

3. Drizzle the olive oil over the salmon and asparagus, and season with salt, pepper, and minced garlic.

4. Arrange the lemon slices on top of the salmon.

5. Bake for 15-20 minutes, or until the salmon is cooked through and the asparagus is tender.

6. Serve the baked salmon and asparagus over a bed of cooked quinoa, and garnish with fresh dill or parsley.

7. Enjoy a nutritious and gut-friendly dinner that is high in protein and omega-3 fatty acids.

2. Gut-Healing Chicken Soup

Ingredients:

1 tablespoon of olive oil

1 onion, chopped

2 cloves garlic, minced

2 carrots, sliced

2 celery stalks, sliced

1 zucchini, chopped

1 cup mushrooms, sliced

1 cup cooked, shredded chicken breast

6 cups chicken broth (preferably homemade or low-sodium)

1 cup of spinach or kale

1 teaspoon dried thyme

1 teaspoon dried rosemary

Salt and pepper to taste

Juice of 1/2 lemon

Instructions:

1. In a large pot, heat the olive oil over medium heat.

2. Add the onion and garlic, and sauté until the onion is translucent.

3. Add the carrots, celery, zucchini, and mushrooms, and cook for about 5 minutes, until the vegetables begin to soften.

4. Stir in the shredded chicken breast and chicken broth.

5. Add the spinach or kale, dried thyme, dried rosemary, salt, and pepper.

6. Bring the soup to a boil, then reduce the heat and simmer for 20–30 minutes.

7. Stir in the lemon juice just before serving.

8. Enjoy a comforting and gut-healing chicken soup that is packed with nutrients and easy to digest.

3. Lentil and Vegetable Stew

Ingredients:

1 tablespoon of olive oil

1 onion, chopped

2 cloves garlic, minced

2 carrots, diced

2 celery stalks, diced

1 red bell pepper, chopped

1 zucchini, chopped

1 cup green or brown lentils, rinsed and drained

4 cups of vegetable broth

1 can (14.5 oz) diced tomatoes

1 teaspoon dried thyme

1 teaspoon dried oregano

1 bay leaf

Salt and pepper to taste

Fresh parsley for garnish

Instructions:

1. In a large pot, heat the olive oil over medium heat.

2. Add the onion and garlic, and sauté until the onion is translucent.

3. Add the carrots, celery, red bell pepper, and zucchini, and cook for about 5 minutes, until the vegetables begin to soften.

4. Stir in the lentils, vegetable broth, diced tomatoes, dried thyme, dried oregano, bay leaf, salt, and pepper.

5. Bring the stew to a boil, then reduce the heat and simmer for 30–40 minutes, or until the lentils are tender.

6. Remove the bay leaf and stir in fresh parsley just before serving.

7. Enjoy a hearty and fiber-rich vegetable stew that supports gut health.

Snacks and Smoothies: Quick and Healthy Options

Healthy snacks and smoothies can help keep your energy levels stable and provide additional gut-friendly nutrients throughout the day. Here are some quick and nutritious options to satisfy your cravings:.

1. Probiotic-Rich Smoothie

Ingredients:

1 cup of plain kefir or probiotic yogurt

1/2 banana

1/2 cup frozen berries

1 tablespoon of chia seeds

1 tablespoon honey or maple syrup (optional)

1/2 teaspoon vanilla extract

Instructions:

1. In a blender, combine the kefir or probiotic yogurt, banana, frozen berries, chia seeds, honey or maple syrup (if using), and vanilla extract.

2. Blend until smooth and creamy.

3. Pour into a glass and enjoy a probiotic-rich smoothie that supports gut health.

2. Veggie Sticks with Hummus

Ingredients:

Carrot sticks

Celery sticks

Cucumber sticks

Bell pepper slices

1 cup hummus (preferably homemade or low-sodium)

Instructions:

1. Prepare the vegetable sticks and arrange them on a plate.

2. Serve with a cup of hummus for dipping.

3. Enjoy a crunchy and fiber-rich snack that promotes good digestion.

3. Gut-Healing Golden Milk

Ingredients:

1 cup unsweetened almond milk or coconut milk

1 teaspoon turmeric powder

1/2 teaspoon ground ginger

1/4 teaspoon ground cinnamon

1 tablespoon of honey or maple syrup

Pinch of black pepper (to enhance turmeric absorption)

Instructions:

1. In a small saucepan, combine the almond milk or coconut milk, turmeric powder, ground ginger, ground cinnamon, honey or maple syrup, and black pepper.

2. Heat the mixture over medium heat, stirring constantly, until it is hot but not boiling.

3. Pour into a mug and enjoy a warm and gut-healing golden milk that supports digestion and reduces inflammation.

4. Chia Seed Pudding

Ingredients:

1/2 cup unsweetened almond milk or coconut milk

2 tablespoons of chia seeds

1 tablespoon of honey or maple syrup

1/2 teaspoon vanilla extract

Fresh berries for topping

Instructions:

1. In a small bowl or mason jar, combine the almond milk or coconut milk, chia seeds, honey or maple syrup, and vanilla extract.

2. Stir well to

combine and ensure the chia seeds are evenly distributed.

3. Cover and refrigerate for at least 2 hours or overnight, until the mixture thickens to a pudding-like consistency.

4. Top with fresh berries just before serving.

5. Enjoy a nutritious and fiber-rich snack that supports gut health.

Chapter 10

Case Studies and Success Stories.

Examining real-life transformations, expert insights, and lessons learnt from these experiences improves our understanding of the impact of gut health on overall well-being significantly. This chapter dives into a variety of case studies and success stories to demonstrate the enormous benefits of having a healthy digestive system. These stories showcase the journeys of people who overcame major health difficulties via dietary adjustments, lifestyle changes, and a dedication to gut health.

Real-Life Transformations

Case Study 1: Sarah's Battle with IBS

Sarah, a 32-year-old marketing professional, had been dealing with Irritable Bowel Syndrome (IBS) for over a decade. Her symptoms included chronic bloating, stomach pain, and irregular bowel movements, which had a severe impact on her quality of life. Despite repeated visits to doctors and various drugs, she saw no relief.

Intervention:
Sarah decided to start a full gut health program with the help of a nutritionist. The program featured:
- Follow a low FODMAP diet to identify and remove trigger foods.
- Introducing probiotics and prebiotics to help balance her gut microbiota.
- Regular exercise and mindfulness methods can help manage stress.

Outcome:
Sarah's symptoms improved significantly within three months. Her bloating and pain subsided, and her bowel motions were more consistent. She also noticed increased energy and a more positive mood. Sarah's story highlights the significance of a personalized approach to gut health that includes both dietary and lifestyle modifications.

Case Study 2: John's Weight Loss Journey

John, a 45-year-old engineer, was diagnosed with both obesity and prediabetes. His doctor cautioned him of the serious health dangers linked with his condition, such as heart disease and type 2 diabetes. John realized he needed to make big lifestyle adjustments but was overwhelmed.

Intervention:
John joined a gut health-focused weight-loss program that included:
a plant-based diet high in fiber, including vegetables, fruits, whole grains, and legumes.
Consume fermented foods regularly, such as yogurt, kefir, and sauerkraut.
Engage in regular physical activity, including aerobic and strength-training exercises.

Outcome:
Over the course of a year, John shed 50 pounds and dramatically improved his blood sugar levels. His cholesterol and blood pressure levels were also stabilized. John's success story emphasizes the importance of gut health in weight management and metabolic wellness.

Case Study 3: Emily's Skin Transformation

Emily, a 27-year-old graphic designer, has had severe acne since she was a teenager. After trying a variety of skincare products and treatments with little results, she began to investigate the relationship between her stomach and skin health.

Intervention:
Emily worked with a holistic dermatologist, who suggested:
removing processed foods and sugar from her diet.
adding a mix of probiotics and prebiotics to help nourish her gut microbiota.
drinking plenty of water and green tea to aid with the detoxification process.

Outcome:
Emily's skin improved dramatically over the course of six months. Her acne cleared up, and her skin became more luminous and even-toned. Emily's story demonstrates how gut health affects skin health and the need to address internal causes for long-term results.

Expert insights and advice.

To shed more light on the relationship between gut health and general well-being, we consult with prominent specialists in the field. These professionals provide helpful advice on gut health and share their findings based on years of work and research.

Dr. Michael Ruscio, DC, is a functional medicine practitioner.

Dr. Ruscio emphasizes the significance of a healthy gut flora in preventing and controlling chronic diseases. He advises his patients to:
Eat a whole-foods diet high in fiber to boost healthy bacteria.
Be cautious of antibiotic use, as it can affect the gut microbiota.
Consider targeted probiotic and prebiotic supplementation, particularly following sickness or antibiotic therapy.

Dr. Robynne Chutkan, MD: Gastroenterologist

Dr. Chutkan, a prominent gastroenterologist, emphasizes the importance of lifestyle variables in gut health. She recommends:
reducing stress with yoga, meditation, and deep breathing exercises.
prioritizing sleep and developing a consistent sleep schedule.
maintaining regular physical exercise, which supports healthy gut motility and microbial diversity.

Kara Landau, RD: Gut Health Dietitian

Kara Landau, a licensed dietitian who specializes in gut health, recommends clients to:

Include a range of plant-based foods to nourish the gut bacteria with fiber and polyphenols.

Stay hydrated; water is necessary for digestion and vitamin absorption.

Monitor food sensitivities and alter their diet accordingly to avoid inflammation and pain.

Lessons Learned and Key Takeaways

Following these case studies and expert perspectives, several significant lessons emerge that can help individuals on their path to better gut health.

1. Personalized approaches produce the best results.

One-size-fits-all solutions are rarely effective when it comes to gut health. Each person's microbiota is unique, as are their nutritional requirements and lifestyle preferences. Tailoring treatments to individual situations offers the best results. Working with healthcare specialists to create a personalized strategy allows you to more effectively address specific difficulties.

2. Diet is fundamental.

A nutrient-dense diet high in fiber, prebiotics, and probiotics is vital for gut health. Consuming a range of fruits, vegetables, whole grains, and fermented foods promotes a diversified and balanced microbiome. Avoiding processed foods, sweets, and bad fats can help avoid intestinal dysbiosis and improve general health.

3. Lifestyle factors matter.

Aside from eating, lifestyle decisions have a significant impact on digestive health. Regular physical activity, appropriate hydration, stress management, and restful sleep are all essential elements. Mindfulness and yoga can help improve gut-brain communication and minimize stress-related digestive disorders.

4. Monitor and adjust.

Keeping note of your nutritional consumption, symptoms, and lifestyle behaviors might provide useful information about what works best for your gut. A gut health notebook can help uncover patterns and triggers, allowing you to make educated changes to your strategy. Regularly monitoring progress with a healthcare provider ensures that any necessary changes are implemented quickly.

5. The Benefits of Probiotics and Prebiotics

Probiotics (good bacteria) and prebiotics (food for these bacteria) are effective strategies for promoting gut health. Probiotic supplements and foods such as yogurt, kefir, and sauerkraut can introduce helpful bacteria, whereas prebiotic fibers found in garlic, onions, and bananas promote their growth.

6. Long-term commitment is key.

Improving and maintaining gut health requires a long-term commitment. Quick fixes are rarely effective, and lasting changes necessitate continual effort and persistence. Adopting a gut-healthy lifestyle can result in long-term benefits to general well-being.

Real-life transformation stories

Mia's Journey to Overcoming Chronic Fatigue.

Mia, a 38-year-old teacher, suffered from persistent weariness and brain fog. Despite proper sleep and a healthy diet, she was continuously weary. She went to a functional medicine practitioner because she suspected she had a stomach problem.

Intervention:
Mia's practitioner suggested:
comprehensive gut testing to detect dysbiosis or

infections.

a customized diet that eliminates common allergens such as gluten and dairy.

Certain supplements, such as probiotics, digestive enzymes, and anti-inflammatory herbs,.

Outcome:

Within six months, Mia's energy levels and mental clarity had significantly improved. Her gut test findings revealed a rebalanced microbiome. Mia's story demonstrates the link between gut health and systemic diseases such as chronic fatigue.

Carlos' Experience with Autoimmune Disease

Carlos, a 50-year-old accountant, was diagnosed with an autoimmune thyroid condition (Hashimoto's thyroiditis). He had symptoms such as weight gain, hair loss, and joint pain. Carlos chose to address his gut health as part of his treatment after learning about its potential role in autoimmune illnesses.

Intervention:

Carlos engaged with a holistic health coach, who led him through:

an elimination diet to detect food allergies.

a program for healing his intestinal lining that includes

vitamins like L-glutamine and zinc.
stress-reduction methods such as tai chi and breathing exercises.

Outcome:

Carlos' symptoms improved dramatically over the course of a year, as did his thyroid function tests. His hair began to regrow, and he shed the extra weight. Carlos' experience emphasizes the importance of gut health in controlling autoimmune diseases.

Conclusion

In this final chapter, we will review the key principles addressed throughout the book, offer encouragement and inspiration to continue your gut health journey, and provide extra resources and references to help your continued efforts. Maintaining a balanced digestive system entails not just treating current symptoms but also promoting long-term health and well-being. Understanding the complexities of gut health enables you to make more educated decisions that will improve your life.

Recap of Key Points

Understanding the Gut

We started by learning about the digestive system's anatomy and how important it is to general health. The gut is a complicated system that includes the mouth, esophagus, stomach, intestines, and other auxiliary organs such as the liver and pancreas. Each component performs specialized duties related to digestion, nutrient absorption, and waste removal.

We also looked into the microbiome, an ecosystem of trillions of bacteria that live in the gut. These bacteria, viruses, fungi, and other microorganisms are essential for digestion, immunity, and even mental wellness. Having a healthy and diversified microbiome is critical for general health.

The gut-brain link was another important topic, as it demonstrated how the gut communicates with the brain via the vagus nerve and other channels. This link affects mood, stress reactions, and cognitive function, emphasizing the significance of a healthy gut for mental health.

Common digestive issues and symptoms

In Chapter 2, we covered a variety of digestive illnesses, including Irritable Bowel Syndrome (IBS), Crohn's disease, ulcerative colitis, and small intestinal bacterial overgrowth. Understanding the causes, symptoms, and potential therapies for these disorders can help you manage and relieve stomach problems.

Recognizing symptoms of an unhealthy gut, such as bloating, gas, constipation, diarrhea, and food intolerances, is critical for early diagnosis and successful management. We also looked into the effects of stress on digestion, underscoring the importance of stress management practices for gut health.

Nutrition for a Healthy Gut

Nutrition is essential for sustaining intestinal health. We talked about how important it is to have a well-balanced diet rich in fiber, vitamins, and minerals. Fruits, vegetables, whole grains, and fermented foods are rich in nutrients and good bacteria, which are essential for a healthy microbiome.

It is equally crucial to understand which meals to avoid. Highly processed foods, extra sweets, and unhealthy fats can disturb gut bacterial balance and cause digestive issues. Making attentive eating choices can benefit your gut health and general well-being.

Probiotics and prebiotics.

Probiotics and prebiotics are vital for gut health. Probiotics are live, helpful bacteria that help balance the gut microbiome. Probiotic-rich foods include yogurt, kefir, sauerkraut, and other fermented goods.

Prebiotics, on the other hand, are fibers that nourish and stimulate the growth of helpful microorganisms. Prebiotic-rich foods include garlic, onions, bananas, and asparagus. Incorporating probiotics and prebiotics into your diet can improve gut health by promoting a healthy microbiome.

Lifestyle changes for improved digestion

Hydration, exercise, and sleep all play an important role in digestion. Drinking enough water helps to break down meals and move waste through the digestive tract. Regular physical activity promotes healthy intestinal motility and lowers stress.

Sleep is another important aspect. Poor sleep has the potential to impair digestion and gut microbial equilibrium. Prioritizing quality sleep and sticking to a consistent sleep schedule can have a big impact on your digestive health.

Healing the gut entails detecting and treating dietary sensitivities and allergies, which can lead to inflammation and other digestive problems. Detoxifying your gut with correct nutrition, water, and toxin avoidance improves overall gut health.

Natural therapies and supplements, such as herbal teas, digestive enzymes, and particular nutrients like L-glutamine, can help the gut heal. These therapies, when combined with a healthy diet and lifestyle adjustments, can help restore and maintain gut health.

The Mind-Gut Connection

The mind-gut connection highlights the impact of mental health on digestion. Stress can exacerbate gut troubles; therefore, stress management practices such as mindfulness and meditation are essential. Mindfulness and regular meditation can help reduce stress and enhance intestinal health.

Developing stress-management skills, such as yoga, deep breathing exercises, and seeking social support, can have a significant impact on mental and digestive health. A peaceful mind promotes a healthy gut, and vice versa.

Personalized Gut Health Plans

Developing a personalized gut health plan entails keeping a gut health notebook to record your nutrition, symptoms, and lifestyle behaviors. Tailoring your food and lifestyle to your particular needs is the most efficient way to preserve gut health.

Long-term gut health techniques include ongoing learning, regular monitoring, and making changes based on your findings and health state. A proactive strategy can lead to long-term improvements in digestive health.

Recipes for Gut Health.

Incorporating gut-friendly dishes into your regular routine can have a huge impact. We included a selection of recipes for breakfasts, lunches, dinners, snacks, and smoothies that are both delicious and beneficial to gut health.

You can nourish your gut and experience the benefits of better digestion and overall health by eating foods that are high in nutrients, fiber, and probiotics.

Case Studies and Success Stories

Real-life transformations and professional insights demonstrated the significant importance of focusing on gut health. Case stories of people who overcame serious health difficulties by changing their diet and lifestyle and committing to gut health are compelling illustrations of what is achievable.

Expert guidance emphasized the significance of tailored methods, a nutrient-dense diet, lifestyle choices, and the benefits of probiotics and prebiotics. These experiences and insights offer invaluable lessons and motivation to anyone on a gut health journey.

Encouragement and Motivation for Your Gut Health Journey

Starting a quest to restore your gut health is an admirable and transformative decision. The route may provide difficulties, but the rewards are tremendous and far-reaching. Below are some crucial areas of encouragement and motivation to help you along the way:

1. Small changes produce big results.

Remember that even minor, gradual improvements can have a major impact over time. You do not have to change your entire lifestyle overnight. Begin with small changes, such as eating more fiber-rich meals, drinking an additional glass of water each day, or adding a short walk to your routine. These little measures can lead to significant health improvements.

2. Listen to your body.

Your body provides useful input on what works and what doesn't. Pay attention to how different foods and lifestyle choices affect your digestion and overall health. Use this knowledge to make informed decisions that benefit your health. Believe that your body understands what it needs.

3. Consistency is key.

Consistency is necessary for long-term change. While it may be tempting to look for quick remedies, long-term health benefits require regular commitment. Stay committed to your gut health strategy, even if improvement appears to be gradual. The advantages will become clearer with time.

4. Celebrate your successes!

Recognize and celebrate your accomplishments, no matter how minor they may appear. Take joy in your accomplishments, whether it's a week of consistent exercise, experimenting with a new gut-friendly recipe, or experiencing fewer symptoms. Celebrating victories increases motivation and promotes good habits.

5. Seek support.

You do not have to go through your gut health journey alone. Seek help from healthcare specialists, nutritionists, or wellness coaches who may offer direction and tailored suggestions. Connect with friends, family, or support groups who have similar health goals. Having a support system can make a big impact.

6. Be patient and compassionate.

Healing and strengthening gut health takes time. Be patient with yourself and accept that setbacks are part of the process. Approach yourself with care, understanding that achieving long-term improvements is a slow process. Every day presents an opportunity to make health-promoting decisions.

7. Stay informed and curious.

Continuing to educate yourself on gut health and general wellness allows you to make more educated decisions. Stay curious and open to learning about new studies, approaches, and strategies that can help you improve your health. Knowledge is an extremely effective tool for maintaining and improving gut health.

Additional resources and references.

Explore the information and references below to help you on your gut health journey. These books, websites, and professional organizations provide useful information, tools, and assistance.

Books

"The Good Gut: Taking Control of Your Weight, Mood, and Long-Term Health" by Justin Sonnenburg and Erica Sonnenburg: This book examines the role of the gut microbiome and provides practical suggestions for improving gut health.

Giulia Enders' "Gut: The Inside Story of Our Body's Most Underrated Organ" is a highly instructive and fascinating book that discusses the gut's complicated activities and how they affect general health.

Dr. Robynne Chutkan's book "The Microbiome Solution: A Radical New Way to Heal Your Body from the Inside Out" provides insights on the microbiome's role in health as well as practical strategies for maintaining a healthy gut.

Websites and online resources

The American Gastroenterological Association (AGA): [gastro.org] (https://www.gastro.org).

The AGA offers extensive information on a variety of digestive problems, treatments, and current research.

The Gut Health Doctor's website is [theguthealthdoctor.com].

Dr. Megan Rossi's website provides evidence-based information, recipes, and resources for better gut health.

National Institute of Diabetes and Digestive and Kidney Diseases (NIDDK): [niddk.nih.gov] (https://www.niddk.nih.gov)

This website provides a wealth of information about

digestive illnesses, including research updates and patient education materials.

Professional organizations and support groups

American Nutritional Association.

(ANA): https://www.theana.org.
The American Nutrition Association promotes nutrition science and offers information for professionals and the general public.
International Scientific Association of Probiotics and Prebiotics (ISAPP): [isappscience.org] (https://www.isappscience.org)
ISAPP provides scientific information about probiotics and prebiotics and their effects on health.
Crohn's and Colitis Foundation: [https://www.crohnscolitisfoundation.org].
This foundation provides assistance, information, and resources to people living with Crohn's disease and ulcerative colitis.

Mobile Applications

Cara Care is a gut health app that allows users to monitor their symptoms, food, and stress levels in order to treat digestive health issues.
MyFitnessPal is a comprehensive nutrition and fitness tracking app that can help you manage your dietary

consumption and promote good eating habits.

Headspace is a meditation and mindfulness app that promotes stress reduction and the mind-gut connection.

Final Thoughts

Starting a gut health journey is a powerful step toward improving your overall health and well-being. You can achieve and maintain a balanced digestive system by understanding the importance of the gut, making smart nutritional choices, adopting healthy lifestyle practices, and getting help when necessary.

This book has equipped you with the knowledge and tools to confidently navigate your gut health journey. Remember that the path to optimal gut health is unique to each person and involves patience, consistency, and a willingness to learn and adapt.

As you progress, stay committed to your health goals, enjoy your accomplishments, and keep learning about new strategies to support your gut. A healthy gut has several benefits beyond digestion, including improved energy levels, mood, immunological function, and general quality of life.

We wish you all the best on your journey to intestinal health and well-being. May the knowledge and insights gained from this book motivate you to make long-term, good changes and live a bright, healthy life.

Appendices

glossary of terms

Antibiotics are medications that treat bacterial infections. While they are efficient at combating infections, they can disturb the gut microbiome by killing beneficial bacteria.

Bloating is a condition in which the abdomen feels full and tight, usually due to gas or other digestive difficulties. It can indicate a number of gut health issues, including dietary intolerances and digestive diseases.

Crohn's disease is a chronic inflammatory bowel disease (IBD) that can affect any region of the gastrointestinal tract, resulting in symptoms such as stomach pain, diarrhea, and weight loss.

Dysbiosis is an imbalance in the microbial community of the gut that is frequently related to health problems such as digestive disorders, allergies, and autoimmune illnesses.

Fermented foods are foods that have undergone fermentation, a process in which natural bacteria feed on sugar and starch to produce helpful probiotics. Examples include yogurt, kefir, sauerkraut, kimchi, and kombucha.

Fiber is a form of carbohydrate that the body can't digest. Fruits, vegetables, whole grains, and legumes all contain it, which is necessary for proper digestion. Fiber regulates the body's usage of glucose, which helps to control hunger and blood sugar levels.

The gut-brain axis is a bidirectional communication network that connects the enteric neural system of the gut to the central nervous system of the brain. This relationship has an impact on mood, stress reactions, and cognitive abilities.

IBS (Irritable Bowel Syndrome) is a common large-intestine illness with symptoms including cramping, stomach pain, bloating, gas, diarrhea, and constipation.

The microbiome is a community of microorganisms, including bacteria, viruses, fungi, and other microbes, that live in a specific environment, such as the human gut. The gut microbiota is crucial for digestion, immunological function, and overall health.

Prebiotics are non-digestible food components, typically fibers, that stimulate the growth of beneficial bacteria in the stomach. Garlic, onions, bananas, and asparagus are among the most common sources.

Probiotics are live bacteria that provide health advantages when taken in suitable doses. They are sometimes referred to as "good" or "friendly" bacteria and are present in fermented foods and nutritional supplements.

SIBO (Small Intestinal Bacterial Overgrowth) is a disorder in which excessive bacteria develop in the small intestine, causing symptoms like bloating, diarrhea, and malnutrition.

Ulcerative colitis is a chronic inflammatory bowel disease (IBD) that mostly affects the colon and rectum, resulting in symptoms such as abdominal pain, diarrhea, and rectal bleeding.

The vagus nerve is the tenth cranial nerve, extending from the brainstem to the belly and controlling the heart, lungs, and digestive tract via the parasympathetic nervous system. It is an essential part of the gut-brain axis.

Recommended reading.

Consider reading the books listed below to learn more about gut health. They provide detailed information, practical recommendations, and evidence-based insights to help you understand and support your journey to better digestive health.

1. Justin and Erica Sonnenburg's book "The Good Gut: Taking Control of Your Weight, Mood, and Your Long-term Health"
This book digs into the science of the microbiome and provides practical recommendations on how to improve your gut bacteria through diet and lifestyle choices.

2. Giulia Enders' book "Gut: The Inside Story of Our Body's Most Underrated Organ"
a fascinating and accessible book that discusses the gut's complicated activities and their impact on general health, written with humor and supported by scientific data.

3. "The Microbiome Solution: A Radical New Way to Heal Your Body from the Inside Out" by Dr. Robynne Chutkan.
This book delves into the microbiome's function in health and provides practical suggestions for maintaining a healthy gut, such as food recommendations and lifestyle advice.

4. Dr. David Perlmutter's "Brain Maker: The Power of Gut Microbes to Heal and Protect Your Brain—For

Life"

Dr. Perlmutter investigates the link between the gut microbiome and brain health, providing dietary and lifestyle recommendations to improve both gut and brain function.

5. "The Clever Gut Diet: How to Revolutionize Your Body From the Inside Out" by Dr. Michael Mosley.

This book offers a thorough guide to improving gut health via dietary changes, with meal plans and recipes that support a healthy microbiome.

6. "The Gut-Immune Connection: How Understanding the Connection Between Food and Immunity Can Help Us Regain Our Health," written by Emeran Mayer

Dr. Mayer investigates the link between the gut and the immune system, providing insights into how dietary choices affect immunological function and overall health.

7. "Fiber Fueled: The Plant-Based Gut Health Program for Losing Weight, Restoring Your Health, and Optimizing Your Microbiome," written by Dr. Will Bulsiewicz

This book stresses the role of dietary fiber and plant-based foods in gut health, and it includes practical advice and recipes for a fiber-rich diet.

8. "The Complete Low-FODMAP Diet: A Revolutionary Plan for Managing IBS and Other Digestive Disorders" by Sue Shepherd and Peter Gibson a step-by-step approach to adopting a low-FODMAP diet, which can help control symptoms of IBS and other digestive diseases by limiting fermentable carbs.

Helpful Websites and Support Groups

Staying informed and connected with individuals who have similar health goals can be really beneficial. The following websites and support groups provide useful information, tools, and communities for gut health and related issues.

Websites

1. The American Gastroenterological Association (AGA)
• [gastro.org](https://www.gastro.org)
The AGA offers extensive information on a variety of digestive problems, treatments, and current research. It is a great resource for both patients and healthcare providers.

2. The Gut Health Doctor
[The Gut Health Doctor](https://www.theguthealthdoctor.com)

Dr. Megan Rossi's website provides evidence-based information, recipes, and resources for better gut health. It comprises articles, blog entries, consultations, and courses.

3. The National Institute of Diabetes, Digestive, and Kidney Diseases (NIDDK)
- [NIDDK.NIH.GOV](https://www.niddk.nih.gov)
This website provides a wealth of information about digestive illnesses, including research updates and patient education materials. It is a reliable source of scientific knowledge about intestinal health.

4. The International Scientific Association for Probiotics and Prebiotics (ISAPP)
• [isappscience.org](https://www.isappscience.org)
ISAPP provides scientific information about probiotics and prebiotics and their effects on health. It provides materials for both researchers and the general public.

5. The Crohn's and Colitis Foundation
Crohnscolitis Foundation (https://www.crohnscolitisfoundation.org).
This foundation provides support, information, and resources to those living with Crohn's disease and ulcerative colitis, such as educational materials and support groups.

6. Global Healing Center
[Global Healing Center] (https://www.globalhealingcenter.com).
a comprehensive source of natural health and wellness information, with articles and products focusing on gut health and detoxification.

7. Precision Nutrition
•[precisionnutrition.com] (https://www.precisionnutrition.com)
Precision Nutrition provides evidence-based articles, programs, and coaching on nutrition and lifestyle modifications to improve overall health, including gut health.

Support Groups

1. IBS Network
[The IBS Network] (https://www.theibsnetwork.org).
a UK-based charity that offers information, support, and resources to those living with Irritable Bowel Syndrome (IBS), including a helpline and online forums.

2. IBD Support Groups
There are several local and online support groups for people with Crohn's disease and ulcerative colitis. These groups offer a place to share experiences, advice, and emotional support. Many IBD support groups meet on websites such as Meetup.com and Facebook.

3. FODMAP-Friendly
•[fodmapfriendly.com]
(htttps://www.fodmapfriendly.com)
This website provides tools and assistance for people on a low-FODMAP diet, including certified low-FODMAP goods and recipes.

4. Gut Health Support Group on Facebook.
a community of people interested in gut health who share advice, recipes, and personal stories. It fosters an environment conducive to discussing gut health concerns and triumphs.

5. Healing Well Community
[healingwell.com/community]
(htttps://www.healingwell.com/community).
an online community that hosts discussions for a variety of health issues, including digestive diseases. It gives a forum for people to discuss their stories, ask questions, and offer assistance to one another.

6. MyGIHealth
Mygihealth.io (https://www.mygihealth.io)
a website and app that provides tools for documenting digestive symptoms, locating educational resources, and engaging with a gut health-focused community.

7. Meetup.com
• [meetup.com](https://www.meetup.com)

a platform for locating local and virtual health and wellness gatherings, such as those focusing on gut health, nutrition, and lifestyle improvements.

Final Thoughts

The path to better gut health is varied, encompassing nutrition, lifestyle modifications, and ongoing learning. The resources in this appendix can help you along the journey by providing helpful information, expert guidance, and a sense of community.

Whether you're reading a new book, visiting an instructive website, or joining a support group, each resource can provide you with the knowledge and encouragement you need to keep your gut healthy. Remember that every journey is unique, and determining the best combination of methods and support is critical to your success. Here's to your continuing health and well-being!

www.ingramcontent.com/pod-product-compliance
Lightning Source LLC
Chambersburg PA
CBHW071210240526
45470CB00018B/1691